Y0-BSR-553

Your PERSONAL TRAINER

THE COMPREHENSIVE GUIDE TO FITNESS & HEALTH

BY
WILLIAM E. KENNAMORE
&
JEFFREY G. RIOPELLE, M.D.

DEMOR PRESS

Copyright © 1998 DEMOR Press (Kennamore & Riopelle). Printed and bound in the United States of America. All rights reserved. No part of this book may be reproduced or transmitted in any form or by any means, electronic or mechanical, including photopying, recording, or by any information storage and retrieval system—except by a reviewer who may quote brief passages in a review to be printed in a magazine or newspaper—without permission in writing from the publisher. For information, please contact DEMOR Press, P.O. Box 393, San Ramon, California 94583

Publisher's Cataloging-in-Publication
(Provided by Quality Books, Inc.)

Kennamore, William E.
    Your personal trainer: the comprehensive guide to fitness, combining physical & mental exercises with current medical facts/William E. Kennamore & Jeffrey G. Riopelle; [Julie Winkelstein, editor; Christina Knapp, illustrator]. --1st ed.
    p.cm.
    Includes index
    Preassigned LCCN: 97-80883
    ISBN: 0-9658906-3-5

    1. Physical fitness. 2. Physical fitness--Nutritional aspects. 3. Stress management. 4. Self-care, Health. I. Riopelle, Jeffrey G. II Title.

RA776.K46 1998   613.7
                              Qb197-41301

Attention Organizations, Exercise Facilities, Healing Centers, and Schools.

Quantity discounts are available on bulk purchases of this book for educational purposes. Special books and book excerpts can also be created to fit specific needs. For information, please contact DEMOR Press, P.O. Box 393, San Ramon, California 94583 or call (510) 757-0112 / FAX (510) 757-1306 / e-mail demor@pacbell.net

THIS BOOK IS DEDICATED TO THOSE SEEKING BALANCE IN THEIR LIVES

Special thanks to my wife Johnna, who supported me mentally and emotionally throughout the writing of this work. I want to thank Bruce Allen who gave us permission to use (What Is A Workout). These ideas have guided me in my efforts to achieve balance in my life. Most importantly I want to thank my co-author, Dr. Jeffrey G. Riopelle, who believed in my ideas. I also want to thank Julie Winkelstein who helped make our words and ideas come to life. Special thanks to Katie Winkelstein-Duveneck, Beth Belzer, Marcus Pierre, Lisa Battagello, Shirley Richards, Dr. Eric Hisaka, Dr. Lori Hamilton, Don Babbitt, Shirley Babbitt, Patrick Costello, Marianne O'Keefe, and Dr. Michael J. Schierman who spent many hours reading the manuscript.

William Kennamore

I'd like to thank my wife Donna, who continues to work supportively by my side and has contributed greatly to my medical knowledge. She has patiently endured the countless weekend hours I've spent over the last four years refining *Your Personal Trainer*. I thank William Kennamore for his original idea of combining our efforts and for his continued dedication to keeping us motivated as we completed our book.

Jeffrey G. Riopelle

TABLE OF CONTENTS

CHAPTER 2—STRENGTHEN YOUR FOUNDATION

CHAPTER 3—CHALLENGE YOURSELF

CHAPTER 4—FIND YOUR ENERGY LEVEL

CHAPTER 7—STAY ON TRACK

CHAPTER 8—STAY HEALTHY AND FIT
AS A WAY OF LIFE

CHAPTER 9—THE EXERCISES

CHAPTER 10—THE REST OF YOUR LIFE

The Order Blank

P R E F A C E

William Kennamore is a certified personal trainer, a credentialed adult health education teacher and an employment enhancement training instructor. He was an Officer in the Marine Corps and has a B.A. degree in psychology, with an emphasis on management. His postgraduate studies have focused on the way in which fitness and health together affect organizational structure and the quality of work that is produced.

William Kennamore's personal training, motivational and employment strategies are all based on his belief that a lifestyle modification must include a complete and ongoing exercise routine, with a constant awareness of the link between body and mind.

Dr. Jeffrey G. Riopelle, a board certified family practitioner, is particularly interested in preventative health maintenance, weight reduction, sports medicine and stress reduction through exercise.

Dr. Riopelle believes wellness is maintained by keeping a balance between physical well-being and contentment with life. In keeping with this, he encourages his patients to ask questions and keep themselves informed, ultimately taking responsibility for their own health.

There are thousands of exercise books and even more diet books. How do you choose the right one for yourself? Maybe the following will help you decide.

"Why did each of you write this book?" our editor asked us. William Kennamore: For myself in answer, I brought out a stack of well-worn notebooks and placed them on my dining room table. Each one of those books represented the time and thoughts one of my many exercise clients had put into his or her own training book. Just as you will keep a diary of your progress in this book, so did they. Each day they recorded what they ate, how they felt, what exercises they did. I guided and supported them, provided them with necessary information, and then watched as they grew more fit.

After working as a personal trainer with more than three thousand clients, I've learned what motivates and what doesn't. I've learned the importance of self-examination as a tool for change, because change without understanding will only lead to failure. There is a connection between your physical state and your mental state. Our book helps you discover this connection for yourself so you can experience a healthier lifestyle. I want to share these techniques.

William E. Kennamore, C.P.T.

A long with William Kennamore, I wrote this book to provide people of all ages with a structured program that teaches the same tools I use for myself and provide for my patients.

When I look at my patients and people in general in today's busy society, I see many good hard working people trying to cope with the pressures of life. I see the toll today's lifestyle can take on one's body. Over the years I've developed methods to help provide optimum physical and mental health that I teach my patients and adhere to myself.

My suggestions include eating well, doing regular stretching, strengthening and aerobic exercises, doing mental relaxation exercises, getting plenty of rest, taking sufficient vacations to recharge one's batteries, and avoiding overindulging in habits that harm one's body.

I also emphasize the connection between daily activities, eating habits and how these affect a person's life. In *Your Personal Trainer* we offer techniques for understanding more about your daily life and how you can incorporate this understanding into a lifelong exercise and health routine. We offer guidance, information and expertise.
The rest is up to you.

Jeff G. Riopelle, M.D.

INTRODUCTION

"How can I improve my attitude, my health and my self-image?"
"How can I start learning ways to make permanent changes, not just
the temporary ones I've made in the past?"

One of the easiest ways to make a positive change in your life is to
begin a structured activity routine. But with so many available, it's
difficult to know which one to choose.

Your Personal Trainer provides exercises, nutrition information,
medical facts and a method of gaining insight into your goals and
obstacles. Each chapter builds on the information and skills you have
acquired.

Our types of exercises were each designed to achieve specific medical
goals. The aerobic exercises increase heart rates, thereby decreasing
risk of heart attack and stroke. They also work muscles repetitively,
thereby burning calories to decrease body fat. The weight resistance
exercises are crucial in helping you maintain a high metabolic rate,
enabling you to burn more calories and again decrease body fat.
The stretching exercises improve body flexibility and decrease the
risk of injury. All three exercise types improve appearance and
improve your sense of well-being.

The medical facts include an understanding of the importance of
cholesterol, hypertension, waist to hip ratio, body fat distribution,
proper nutritional intake and the avoidance of smoking as well as
many other topics. We have covered common medical ailments of
depression and anxiety, including prevention and treatments. We have
discussed screening and prevention of heart attacks, stroke and various
preventable cancers. Additionally, we have discussed numerous common medical disorders such as diabetes, hypothyroidism, arthritis and
fibromyalgia. In regards to obesity, there is an overview of newer
advances in the understanding of the causes of obesity and medications
for treatment.

The written exercise portions of *Your Personal Trainer* focus on ways to improve your emotional well-being, since it is our belief that how you think and feel plays a major role in prevention of medical disorders.

Your Personal Trainer teaches you how to get started in an exercise routine and how to stay with it. Step by step, day by day, you will learn techniques to increase your energy, think positively and feel good about yourself. These techniques are designed to help you change old habits into new and positive lifestyle behaviors.

With the current interest in physical and leisure activities, many people have become aware of the importance of daily exercise combined with careful nutrition. Yet, seven out of the ten leading causes of death in the United States are due to lifestyle behaviors. These behaviors are linked to coronary heart disease, hypertension, obesity, chronic fatigue and depression. Few people actually find a solution for permanent change.

Over the last ten years we have seen an increase in the number of people using physical activities, such as sports or individual exercise, to improve their lifestyle. At the same time, the medical community has told us we should also concentrate our attention on the food we consume and the way we conduct our lives. None of us wants to become a statistic of Syndrome X: hyperlipidemia, adult onset diabetes or obesity leading to coronary artery disease and stroke. Our lifestyles also increase the risk of life-threatening cancers, especially cancers of the lung, breast, stomach and colon. Along with these physical manifestations come stress and depression. Ten to thirty percent of our population will suffer significant depression or chronic anxiety during his/her lifetime.

How can we reduce these health risks brought on by our lifestyles, or simply improve our self-image, appearance and general health?
We provide an informative and active step-by-step approach that will teach you how to make permanent lifestyle changes. All of this is in *Your Personal Trainer*. As you are about to begin, we encourage you to have patience with yourself and faith in your ability to achieve your goals. This book is for you.

QUESTIONS ABOUT EXERCISE:

Q. I've been thinking about starting an exercise program, but I'm finding it difficult to choose one. How is your book different from others?

A. It's true that there are many programs available, for both losing weight and becoming more fit. Short-term, you may acheive these goals, but without understanding how and why, the results probably won't last. Our book offers something different. We see physical fitness as a means to developing mental fitness. While observing your feelings you will learn to set a goal for yourself, then persevere and accomplish that goal.

Q. How does your program do this?

A. Each chapter in this book has a goal. These include:
1. **Body awareness:** Your measurements, training heart rate, eating habits, sleeping habits, relationships, endurance and any health problems you may have can all affect your ability to take care of yourself.

2. **Learning to trust yourself and your exercise program:** To be successful, you must believe in what you're doing.

3. **Overcoming myths:** Learning the facts about exercise, nutrition and health.

4. **Your wishes:** Understanding what motivates you.

5. **Time:** Learning to organize your daily time in a way that is efficient yet comfortable. Examining areas where you feel out of control.

Q. If I'm a beginner who hasn't exercised in the last 6 to 12 months or who is exercising for the first time, why is it important to follow the first 3 weeks of Your Personal Trainer?

A. The first 3 weeks will help you establish a fitness foundation. The first 3 weeks will also help you make the physical and mental adjustments associated with physical effort. Without this foundation, it's difficult to move on in your exercise program. These include:

1. Taking your measurements
2. Preparing yourself with the necessary equipment
3. Choosing a place to workout
4. Making daily entries in your book
5. Learning to stretch
6. Stocking your kitchen with appropriate food
7. Keeping a diary of your daily eating habits
8. Getting massages
9. Taking quiet time for yourself
10. Self-awareness

Q. If I feel that I might have trouble working on my own through Your Personal Trainer's book, would you recommend hiring a trainer to help me?

A. Yes, some people may get the best help from this book by doing it in conjunction with a trainer.

Q. If I need someone to help me, what are the most important qualities to look for in a trainer?

A. Find someone who is:
1. **Knowledgeable**, about equipment, exercises, training, & nutrition
2. **Supportive**, understanding about your individual needs
3. **Safety Conscious**, about proper alignment
4. **Compatible**, easy for you to be with
5. **Encourages**, questions and provides logical answers

6. **Motivating,** believes in a lifelong routine
7. **Energetic,** stamina is at a level you feel comfortable
8. **Sensible,** knows when to push and when to let up
9. **Experienced,** good reference from clients, other trainers or a physician, and longevity in the industry
10. **Credible,** certified by the state, keeps current
11. **Flexible,** their schedule fits yours
12. **Realistic,** about your body type, state of mind and goals that you have and amount of time in which they can be achieved
13. **Committed,** to training with you until you feel comfortable on your own
14. **A Good Communicator and Listener,** relays information but at the same time listens to your fears and complaints
15. **A Good Teacher,** can explain information in an easily understood way
16. **Professional** regarding manners and attitude
17. **Enjoys Their Work,** shows a genuine interest and love for what they do

HIRING A PERSONAL TRAINER:

1. *How many years should a trainer be working as a trainer before I hire him/her?*
   At least a year, preferably more.

2. *How did the trainer get started in his/her work?*
   Through a combination of classroom training, book work and personal experiences.

3. *How long does the trainer recommend you stay with him/her as a client?*
   It will depend on your goals. It's important that the trainer encourage your eventual independence. Remember, if you are looking for some one just to teach you, eight weeks should be enough time.

However, if you are looking for a partner or someone to motivate you, time can be extended.

4. *What is the trainer's success rate?*
At least 80% of clients are satisfied with their techniques.

5. *How does the trainer structure a normal program?*
The best program is structured with cardiovascular exercises early in each session as a warm-up. Then, if you are a beginner,strengthening and stretching each muscle group should follow.
For example, a program may start with a 20-40 minute aerobic warm-up, then quad strengthening followed by quad stretch then on to hamstring strengthening and hamstring stretch and so on. More advanced programs should still start with aerobic warm-ups, but the strengthening and stretching can vary.

6. *How much does it cost?*
The training per hour may vary depending on whether you want a trainer from a club/gym or you want one that is independent. The average cost can range from 30 – 80 dollars per hour.

7. *Does the trainer monitor heart rate before, during and after the workout?*
Yes, it's important to know how your heart is functioning while you are working out. If you have a trainer working with you, it is important that he/she be constantly aware of your heart rate.

8. *If I start having pain, what should a trainer do?*
It depends on the type of pain. For minor joint pain, stop the activity, apply ice and rest the joint. For muscular pain, stretch and/or massage the area. For minor back or neck pain, stop the exercise and ice and rest the area. For chest pain or any other debilitating pain, stop and see your physician.

9. *How many references should a trainer provide?*
Make sure that you get at least five names. Call at least three.

HOW TRAINERS CAN USE THIS BOOK:

Trainers can use *Your Personal Trainer* to complement their training program, guiding their client through each section. The written portions of the book can be done independently or with the trainer.

Having the support of a personal trainer while learning more about nutrition, exercise and physiology can only enhance the effects of this book.

DISCLAIMER

Your Personal Trainer provides an informed and active approach to preventative health and fitness. This is a guide to improving your way of life and cardiovascular fitness and may, in turn, help reduce risks of diseases associated with the heart and other physical and mental functions. However, various individuals may respond differently to our suggestions. Therefore, we can make no guarantees that everyone will have success using them. The level of success will vary depending on who you are and your degree of motivation.

As with any recommended lifestyle modification routine using physical workouts, you should have the clearance of your physician prior to starting. Some exercises outlined in this book may be too strenuous for individuals with previous injuries or with any preexisting medical condition, such as arthritis. Consult your physician regarding tolerance for these exercises. Also, mild discomfort during exercise and mild soreness and stiffness the following day are normal. However, should you experience more severe pain during or after any specific exercise, stop the activity and consult your physician.

This book is derived from a combination of current medically supported research and our own anecdotal experiences working with patients and physical fitness clients. We have used this program with more than three thousand clients.

GET STARTED

CHANGE YOUR ATTITUDE

LEARN TO THINK IN A NEW WAY

Once you have decided you want to change some of your old habits, you must learn to think in a new way. This new thinking will help you cope with the many obstacles you may have encountered in the past as you tried to change your lifestyle patterns. To create new habits, you must not only be committed to change, but must be prepared for the normal resistance all of us feel.

You may have tried other lifestyle change programs or exercise routines and given up. You may have reached a particular goal and then stopped, eventually finding yourself back where you started. By following this program you will gain confidence and the ability to achieve physical and mental fitness. As you reach the goals you have set for yourself, you will learn how to make a healthy lifestyle a permanent part of your life.

You will learn how to:

- Believe in yourself and the techniques you are using

- Persist even when change is slow

- Take care of yourself

- Think independently

Change is difficult, for everyone. Developing new habits and feeling comfortable with them is an essential part of the adjustment. This book will guide you through this transition and keep you motivated. The routine emphasizes consistency and repetition, so that your mind and your body have a chance to learn new behaviors and replace old ones. We will teach you how to recognize and overcome thoughts which have hindered you in the past. It is natural to feel overwhelmed or unsure when starting a new life change routine. *Your Personal Trainer* will help you examine these feelings and move past them to a healthy and fit way of life.

MOTIVATION

There may have been times in your life when you have felt the effort
to do anything was too much. You had difficulty concentrating, maybe
had sleep disturbances, headaches or back pains. In order to cope with
these feelings, you may have started or increased the use of alcohol or
drugs. You may have started overeating or stopped eating. The final
result of all this can be a tendency to alternate between feeling positive
about yourself and feeling anxious, maybe even phobic. Motivation is
an essential part of any program that will change and improve your
life. But there are two kinds of motivation. *Your Personal Trainer* will
help you discover where your motivation starts and how to guide
yourself in a way that will keep you moving toward your goals.

EXTERNAL MOTIVATION

Many people find it necessary to have a list of shoulds'. They find
themselves saying: I should exercise, I should eat less, I should control
my temper. But should come from outside of us, either to please others
or to live up to some idea of how we feel we ought to be. Feeling you
should exercise may get you started, but as you may have already
discovered, it won't be enough to keep you going. When change is not
prompted by truly wanting to be different, there may be one of two
possible results. Feeling pressured and with weakening motivation,
you quit and feel as if you've failed. Or, you reach a goal, and, re-
lieved, return to your previous habits. Either way, you haven't made
exercise and good health a permanent way of life.

INTERNAL MOTIVATION

Just as it sounds, internal motivation comes from within. This kind of
motivation follows naturally when you reach the point where you want
change. You want to be healthier or thinner or more relaxed, not
because you think it would be a good idea, but because you know your
life would be better. This "desire" will start the process and establish a
guide towards permanent change. It will maintain you as you encounter the natural barriers to making your life different.

**Sometimes it's difficult to put our wants into words.
Following is a list of possible wants.
Check the ones that apply to you or add your own.**

☐ *I want to be in charge of my life.*

☐ *I want how I appear and how I feel to match the mental picture
I have of myself.*

☐ *As I get older, I want to stay healthy and energetic.*

☐ *I want to be more accepting of myself.*

☐ *I want to feel proud of my appearance.*

☐ *I want to feel proud of my accomplishments.*

☐ *I want to enjoy my life and feel happy with what I have.*

☐ *I want to be self-motivated and not need to compare myself to others.*

☐ *I want to feel less tense.*

☐ *I want to take hikes and not be exhausted.*

☐ *I want to have energy and stamina.*

☐ *I want to move gracefully.*

☐ *I want my own character and style to come through.*

☐ *I want boldness and conviction in my walk.*

☐ *I want muscle tone and vitality.*

☐ *I want to have dreams and goals.*

☐ *I want to face my life with optimism, not depression.*

☐ *I want good friends.*

☐ *I want serenity and peace instead of anxiety.*

☐ *I want to know myself.*

☐ *I want to feel and look confident.*

☐ *I want to be healthier and more fit than my parents.*

☐ *I want to look forward to my workouts.*

☐ *I want to tone my body and lose some weight.*

☐ *I want the time to adjust to major changes in my life,
    such as surgery, a new job, money problems, a death in the family.*

**Did you find some of your wants on this list?
Our book can help you find your motivation,
understand the obstacles and succeed.**

GET STARTED

Before you begin your new routine, we will help you lay a foundation of healthful habits.

THIS FOUNDATION WILL INCLUDE:

- Examining the obstacles in your path to physical and mental fitness and looking at solutions for removing them

- Taking a realistic look at your body

- Listing your starting goals

- Taking a look at your eating patterns

- Understanding your metabolism

- Analyzing your time schedule and setting up time goals for yourself

- Finding your target heart rate

- Understanding risk factors

- Overcoming myths about fitness and exercise

The first task is to determine what your approach to physical fitness has been.

Are you a person who hasn't exercised in the last twelve months (or longer) or hasn't ever been on a structured physical fitness routine in your life?

Are you a person who starts with good intentions but doesn't maintain a routine long enough to achieve your goals?

Are you a person who has exercised regularly but wants to make changes in your old routine? Do you sometimes exercise or follow a radical nutritional formula to excess?

KNOW YOUR HEALTH AND FITNESS OBSTACLES

If any of the above descriptions fit you, *Your Personal Trainer* can help you help yourself to change. Sometimes, no matter what you want to accomplish, you may let obstacles block your way. By carefully examining how this happens, you can keep yourself moving in the direction you want to go. The following questions will give you an opportunity to see what is stopping you and how you can get help.

Circle the answer that fits you best and fill in the blank when asked. After each obstacle example, list a possible solution to the obstacle.

Do family responsibilities keep you from being healthy and fit?
     Yes   *No*   *Sometimes*

How many days a week do you devote to physical fitness?

List the types of responsibilities that keep you from physical fitness.
e.g: I have my children with me when I'm not working.

    1.

    2.

    3.

Is lack of family support a major reason why you have not started or maintained a health and fitness routine?
     Yes   *No*   *Sometimes*

How can family members support you in starting or maintaining your routine?
e.g: My husband could drop off the kids at school, so I could get up early and go to work out.

    1.

    2.

    3.

Do you find it hard to get to a workout facility because of work or other responsibilities?
     Yes   *No*   *Sometimes*

Can you invest in workout equipment?   *Yes   No*
e.g: Organize a room or your garage.

    1.

    2.

    3.

Do other people have a negative effect on how much you exercise?
    Yes   No   Sometimes

Explain what you could do to overcome these effects.
e.g: I could do more physical activities with my friends, such as going to the gym or taking a walk, instead of going out to eat.

    1.

    2.

    3.

Is not having enough time a major reason you don't participate in physical fitness activities as much as you would like?
    Yes   No   Sometimes

Explain how you could gain more time to participate in a physical fitness activity each week.
e.g: I could walk or bicycle every day at lunch time.

    1.

    2.

    3.

Is it easier for you to workout at home?
    Yes   No   Sometimes

Explain what you can do to set up your workouts at home.
e.g: Buy the equipment I need and workout at home.

    1.

    2.

    3.

The items below are other obstacles you may encounter when you try to start or maintain a physical fitness routine. We have discussed some of these already. After reading the list, add any you feel should be included. Then rank them from most (1) to least (14 or higher) likely to prevent you from reaching your goal.

- Time
- Cost
- Lack of family support
- Fatigue
- Inconvenience
- Knowing what to do
- Work

- Family responsibilities
- Pain/discomfort
- Embarrassment
- Lack of proper facilities
- Weather
- Transportation
- Other people

Notice the top three. Can you think of solutions for these? Write your ideas here:

1.

2.

3.

As you begin this new lifestyle, remember these three obstacles and their solutions. To remind yourself, fill out the personal agreement below and display it so you will see it every day.

MY PERSONAL AGREEMENT

> *I hereby promise myself I will not let these three obstacles prevent me from maintaining my lifestyle change routine. These are:*

1.

2.

3.

BODY AWARENESS
One of the motivations for starting and maintaining a physical fitness routine is the desire to look different. But it's important to be realistic about your goals.

WHICH BODY TYPE ARE YOU:
An **ectomorph** has a thin, light bone structure and long tenuous muscles. Fat retention isn't a problem, but developing large muscle mass is very difficult.

A **mesomorph** has the capacity for quickly becoming muscular. Fat retention can become a problem, but can be controlled with exercise.

An **endomorph,** has thick bones and a general tendency to be stocky or round. Endomorph will have more difficulty developing muscle tone, so their main goal will be to lose fat.

Even though there are these three basic types, most people are combination of body types. For instance, you could be:

An endo-meso, with the capacity to develop a muscular look, but also needing to be concerned with fat retention.

An ecto-meso, with the capacity to develop a muscular look, but without the problem of fat retention.

Knowing more about your body type will help you to develop realistic goals and recognize the progress you have made. Combining this information with the proper nutritional choices will give you the most effective health and fitness routine.

STARTING GOALS

Committing yourself to a new and healthy way of life includes more than just physical fitness and eating well. It's also an opportunity to examine your whole life and see where you want other changes to occur. For each category, take the time to examine your daily life and assess what you want to improve. Then, write down three changes you would like to make.

MENTAL
e.g. One hour reading daily

a.
b.
c.

PHYSICAL
e.g. One hour exercise

a.
b.
c.

WORK
e.g. Maintain a high standard

a.
b.
c.

STRESS RELEASE
e.g. Get a monthly
        massage

a.
b.
c.

NUTRITIONAL
e.g. Learn to eat for good health

a.
b.
c.

TIME
e.g. Set up a daily
      schedule

a.
b.
c.

RELATIONSHIPS
e.g. Be more assertive

a.
b.
c.

EDUCATION
e.g. Learn computer skills

a.
b.
c.

LIFE EVENTS

e.g. Recognize the negative and
      enjoy the positive

a.
b.
c.

MONEY

e.g. Set up a saving plan

a.
b.
c.

EATING PATTERNS

To better understand the choices you make in foods and the times you eat, it's helpful to be aware of what you are thinking and feeling before, during and after you eat. Keep this record as a part of your daily routine. To get you started, answer these questions for one forty-eight hour period. As you progress with *Your Personal Trainer*, keep these questions in mind.

An hour before eating:
What are you thinking about and how do you feel?

While you are eating:
What are you thinking about and how do you feel?

Two hours after eating:
What are you thinking about and how do you feel?

Four hours after your last meal:
What are you thinking about and how do you feel?

How you are feeling and what you are thinking about before, during and after you eat all play an important role in your eating patterns. The amount of time is also important. There will be more about this later. First, let's look at three areas of your activities. To consider your daily calorie needs, the day can be divided into three time periods: work/school, sleep, leisure and other activities. During each period you will need to eat a percentage of your daily calorie needs.

The following table gives these periods and the percentages for each.

ACTIVITY	AVERAGE HOURS	% OF DAILY CALORIES
Sleep	8	15
Work and/or school	8	45
Leisure and other activities	8	40
Totals per day	*24*	*100*

When considering how to space your meals and snacks during the hours while you're awake, keep these rules in mind:

Eat every two hours if you want to gain weight

Eat every three hours if you want to maintain your weight

Eat every four hours if you want to lose weight

Five hours or more between meals will put you in food deprivation

An easy way to remember this is with this rhyme:

Two to gain
Three to maintain
Four to lose
&
Five to abuse

EXAMINE YOUR APPROACH TO EXERCISE
There are four fitness types: Beginner, Ambivalent, Obsessive and Balanced. Which are you?

BEGINNER
In exercise, a beginner is a person who has decided to start an exercise routine or a person who has not worked out in the last twelve months. If you are a beginner, it's important for you to gather as much information as possible. Initially, it may be a good investment to hire a personal motivator to teach and motivate you. Follow the directions in this book carefully, giving yourself the opportunity to not only learn but experience a healthy lifestyle. As a beginner, be sure you have:

- Accurate information
- Precise directions

AMBIVALENT
An ambivalent exerciser has conflicting emotions and thoughts about whether it's worth the benefits to workout or the effort it takes to do the work. If you're ambivalent about exercising, guilt probably plays a role in your daily life. You can learn to take advantage of this feeling. When you start to feel guilty, look at the situation. What can you do for yourself? If you don't feel like exercising, decide to do it anyway. Choose an activity you enjoy, to make it as easy as you can for yourself. Then, when you've finished, notice how you feel. Another way to get beyond ambivalence or resistance is to exercise with a partner. Working out with someone else helps you stay motivated and focused and can help you look forward to your exercise time. As an ambivalent exerciser, be sure you:

- Use guilt to your advantage
- Consider working out with a partner
- Choose an exercise you enjoy

OBSESSIVE

An obsessive exerciser's effort is extreme. If you are obsessive about exercise, your biggest challenge is to lessen your intensity. Exercise is important, but it shouldn't prevent you from keeping your commitments. You shouldn't push yourself so hard that you injure yourself. Remember, a healthy lifestyle is more than exercise. It's a balance of nutrition, exercise, self-awareness and relaxation. Without any one of these components you will eventually quit your routine.

As an Obsessive exerciser, remember to:

- Keep perspective to prevent obsession

- Take time for yourself in ways other than exercising

BALANCED

A balanced exerciser understands that it's important to work for equilibrium in his or her life. As a balanced exerciser, you have learned moderation. You exercise and eat well, but not compulsively. You choose activities you enjoy and know you will pursue, so you don't need to feel guilty. You exercise with a partner if you want to, knowing a companion can make your exercise time more enjoyable. You stay informed, motivated and self-aware as much as possible, and that's enough. As a balanced exerciser, you understand:

- The importance of equilibrium within your life

- The importance of moderation in exercise and eating

- How to stay informed, motivated and self-aware

This book is designed to help all fitness types. We provide structure and the opportunity to challenge yourself, no matter what type you are. If you are a beginner, you will have the information you need and the opportunity to form proper exercise habits. If you're an ambivalent exerciser, the structure and variety will keep you moving. An obsessive exerciser will find the self-examination as important as the structure.

UNDERSTANDING YOUR METABOLISM

Your body uses the foods you eat as fuel for energy. Fats, proteins and carbohydrates are all used as fuel. The energy values of these foods are:

1 gram carbohydrate=4 calories

1 gram protein=4 calories

1 gram fat=9 calories

Looking at these numbers, you can easily see that fats, with the most calories, also give you the most energy. But you must look at the quality of that energy. That is, the kind of calories you are consuming. The quality and quantity of calories you are consuming will determine whether you gain, lose or maintain your weight. They will also affect how you feel. One of the difficulties in choosing the correct foods is that most people tend to eat the foods that taste best to them. This may lead to eating more high calorie foods and subsequently to unwanted weight gain and low energy levels. But as you get to know more about your body and how you feel eating well and exercising regularly, you will find yourself choosing foods more carefully. To begin this process, we will start with your Basal Metabolic Rate (BMR). Your BMR is the amount of energy required to sustain your body while you are at rest, lying down. In the average adult, this number is about 1400 calories per day for women and 1800 calories per day for men.

However, many factors influence your BMR. These include age, size, lifestyle, body composition and heredity. Most important to remember is that when you increase your activity level, you increase your need for energy. Some of the results of this fact are:

- More energy is required to maintain muscle tissue built up through exercise.

- Less energy is required to maintain fat cells.

- More calories are burned during exercise.

- Your metabolic rate during walking is twice that of sitting.

- Running uses three times as much energy as walking.

- Climbing stairs uses twice as much energy as running.

- When you are under a great amount of stress, more calories are required than usual.

It's important to remember that when you consume food, over seventy percent of the energy from that food is used to keep your vital processes, such as heart and brain, operating. The remaining thirty percent is used for daily activities. There are three different energy sources: fats, protein and carbohydrates. The daily proportions of each should generally be: 50% carbohydrate, 35% protein and 15% fat. But to know how many grams of each of these you require, you must know the correct calorie count for your age, activity level, sex and weight. Also, you must include information as to whether you want to lose weight, gain weight or maintain your weight.

For example:

If you are on a workout routine that includes an equal amount of aerobic training (30 minutes) and weight training (30 minutes), take in 40% carbs and 40% proteins, with 20% fats. If you are balancing aerobic with anaerobic workouts it's a good idea to balance your intake.

If you are on a workout routine that includes more aerobic training (40-50 minutes) than weight training (10-15 minutes), take in 50% carbohydrates and 30% proteins, with 20% fats. If you are doing more aerobic training than anaerobic training, it's a good idea to take in more carbohydrates in order to have the necessary amount to perform the exercise.

If you are on a workout routine with more weight training (40-50 minutes) than aerobic training (10-15 minutes) take in 50% proteins and 30% carbohydrates, with 20% fats. If you are doing more anaerobic training, it's a good idea to take in more proteins because proteins help build muscle. Remember these are examples. They may vary depending on the intensity of your workouts and whether you are trying to lose weight. If you have significant amounts of weight to lose, lower your fat intake to10% and increase your carbohydrates by 10%.

RULES FOR HEALTHY EATING:
Once you know the calories you should be taking in, read the following to decide where and how you will get them to supply your body with the necessary energy. As you learn to balance your intake of carbohydrates, protein and fat, you may find yourself wanting to stay with just a few safe foods. But to make this a lifetime commitment, rather than a temporary way of eating, follow these four rules.

RULE 1 EAT AN ASSORTMENT OF FOODS.
This will give you variety, as well as increasing your chances of receiving the full range of vitamins and minerals.

RULE 2 EVERY DAY, EAT FOODS FROM ALL FOOD SOURCES
These include milk, meat, fruits, vegetables and grains. If for personal or physical reasons you don't eat from all of these groups, eat from as many as possible.

Dairy products/Eggs
0-fat, 1% or low-fat milk, buttermilk, evaporated or powered, low-fat yogurt with less than 6 gm. of fat per ounce egg whites, cholesterol-free egg substitutes

Beef, poultry, fish
Lean cuts of meat with fat trimmed, chicken and turkey without skin, white fish

Fruits and vegetables
Fresh, frozen, canned or dried fruits and vegetables

Breads, cereals, pasta, rice, dried peas and beans
Most breads, bagels, muffins, rice cakes, low-fat crackers, hot and cold cereals, spaghetti, macaroni, noodles, whole grain rice, dried peas and beans

Fats and Oils (No more than 8 teaspoons per day)
Safflower, corn, olive, soybean, peanut and, canola oils, margarine

Snacks (Stay away from prepackaged and sweets)
Sherbet, sorbet, frozen yogurt, fruit juices, tea and coffee, hard candy, fig bars, popcorn, pretzels

RULE 3 EAT THESE FOODS IN MODERATION

When you practice moderation, you'll be able to get the nutrients you need without adding unnecessary calories.

Dairy products/Eggs
2% milk, cheese, lite cream cheese or sour cream/egg yolks
(less than 3 per week)

Breads, cereals, pasta, rice, dried peas and beans
Pancakes, waffles, biscuits, muffins and cornbread

Fats and Oils:
Nuts, seeds, avocados, olives

Snacks:
Ice milk, fruit crisps and cobblers, homemade cakes and pies prepared with unsaturated oils

RULE 4 ABSTAIN FROM FOODS WHICH ARE HIGH IN FAT

The following foods should be avoided as much as possible. Although they may taste good, they are not good for you.

Beef, poultry, fish:
Meats with fatty cuts, sausage, bacon or regular packaged luncheon meats

Dairy products:
Whole milk, cream, half & half, imitation products, whipped cream, custard-style yogurt, hard cheese traditional cream cheese or sour cream

Fats and Oils:
Butter, bacon fat, lard, coconut and palm kernel oil

Breads, cereals, pasta, rice, dried peas and beans:
Croissants, sweet rolls, danishes, doughnuts and crackers made with saturated oils, egg noodles, pasta and rice prepared with cream, butter or cheese sauces

Vegetables:
Vegetables prepared in butter, cream or sauce

Snacks:

> Ice cream, frozen tofu, candy, chocolate, potato chips, buttered popcorn, milkshakes, floats, eggnog, store bought pies, frosted pound cakes

HOW TO SELECT YOUR FOOD INTAKE:

As you see it's important that you eat from all food sources, eat an assortment of foods and do it in moderation. Now, let's look at how to structure your nutritional intake during the hours while you're awake. Remember, if you want to gain weight eat every two hours, if you want to maintain your weight eat every three hours, if you want to lose weight eat every four hours and if you go over five or more hours without eating you will harm yourself.

The following are a list of nutritional plans that can be used in conjunction with your workouts. Keep in mind that all of the food items can be substituted with other low fat items of your choosing. It's important when following these nutritional schedules to eat at consistent times and maintain moderate portions. Moderation is the key not only with food consumption but every aspect in your life. So eat healthfully and use different spices and herbs to make your food more exciting. These are life long eating habits that you are establishing. In each directive proteins, carbohydrates and fats are listed in grams.

NUTRITIONAL DIRECTIVE 1

Breakfast:	Amount	CAL	PRO	CARB	FAT
lowfat milk	1 cup	80	8	12	traces
cereal	1 cup	140	4	30	0
piece of fruit	1 med	80	0	20	0
Totals		**300**	**12**	**63**	**traces**

1st Snack:	Amount	CAL	PRO	CARB	FAT
Sandwich of	1/2				
poultry, or tuna	1 oz.	55	7	0	3
Wheat bread	2 slices	140	4	30	0
Mayo, lowfat	2 tsp.	45	0	0	5
Lettuce & Tomato	1 cup	50	4	10	0
Totals		**290**	**15**	**40**	**8**

Lunch:	Amount	CAL	PRO	CARB	FAT
Yogurt	1 cup	80	8	12	traces
Cottage Cheese	1 cup	80	8	12	traces
Totals		**160**	**16**	**24**	**traces**

2nd Snack:	Amount	CAL	PRO	CARB	FAT
Sandwich of	1/2				
poultry or tuna	1 oz.	55	7	0	3
Wheat bread	2 slices	140	4	30	0
Mayo, lowfat	2 tsp	45	0	0	5
Lettuce & Tomato	1 cup	50	4	10	0
Totals		**290**	**15**	**40**	**8**

Dinner:	Amount	CAL	PRO	CARB	FAT
Poultry, fish, steak beef < 15% fat	4 oz	220	28	0	12
Broccoli, squash Zucchini, Spinach or Cauliflower	1 Cup	25	2	5	0
Baked potato	1 med	140	4	30	0
Citrus juices	2 cups	80	0	20	0
Totals		**465**	**34**	**55**	**12–15**

Day's Totals		**1505**	**92**	**222**	**25–30**

NUTRITIONAL DIRECTIVE 2

Breakfast:	Amount	CAL	PRO	CARB	FAT
lowfat milk	1/2 cup	40	4	6	traces
oatmeal	1 cup	140	4	30	0
piece of fruit	1 med	80	0	20	0
Totals		**260**	**8**	**56**	**traces**

1st Snack:	Amount	CAL	PRO	CARB	FAT
Sandwich of	1/2				
poultry, or tuna	1 oz.	55	7	0	3
Wheat bread	2 slices	140	4	30	0
Mayo, lowfat	2 tsp	45	0	0	5
Lettuce & Tomato	1 cup	50	4	10	0
Totals		**290**	**15**	**40**	**8**

Lunch:	Amount	CAL	PRO	CARB	FAT
Yogurt	1 cup	80	8	12	traces
Piece of fruit	1 med	80	0	20	0
Totals		**160**	**8**	**32**	**traces**

Dinner:	Amount	CAL	PRO	CARB	FAT
Poultry, fish, steak beef < 15% fat	4 oz	220	28	0	12
Broccoli, squash Zucchini, Spinach or Cauliflower	1 Cup	25	2	5	0
Baked potato	1 med	140	4	30	0
Citrus juices	2 cups	80	0	20	0
Totals		**465**	**34**	**55**	**12–15**
Day's Totals		**1175**	**65**	**183**	**15–20**

TAKING A CLOSER LOOK AT YOUR DAILY TIME SCHEDULE

Your Personal Trainer will help you change old unhealthy habits to healthy and fit ones. Before you can do this, you must take a close look at all aspects of your life that could interfere with this change. We have looked at some of the obstacles you may encounter while establishing a fit and healthy routine.

Finding the time in your schedule may seem like one of the most insurmountable tasks. However, with a little planning you can meet this challenge. To begin finding this time, it's essential to first see when and how you are currently organizing your day. So begin by answering the following questions:

1._____ How much time do you spend sleeping?

2._____ How much time do you spend in bed before getting up?

3._____ How much time do you spend eating breakfast?

4._____ How much time does it take to leave the house for work/school/other?

5._____ How much time do you spend getting to work/school or other?

6._____ How much time do you spend at work/school/other?

7._____ How much time do you spend eating lunch?

8._____ How much time do you spend working out?

9._____ How much time do you spend getting home from work/school/other?

10._____ How much time do you spend eating dinner?

11._____ How much time do you spend with your family/friends?

12._____ How much time do you spend watching television?

13._____ How much time do you spend for your own quiet time?

14._____ How much time do you spend studying for work assignments?

15._____ How much time do you spend for pleasure reading?

16._____ How much time do you devote to chores?

17._____ What time do you go to bed?

Look back over this schedule. Do you have enough time for everything you want to do? Are there changes you would like to make? List the activities that need more time. I want to create time for the following:

1.

2.

3.

4.

5.

6.

7.

*As you progress through **Your Personal Trainer,** you will be shown how to coordinate all of your personal goals: emotional, physical, nutritional, and time management. With this overall approach, you will have a chance to live a more energetic and healthy life.*

MONITORING YOUR HEART RATE

As you begin to work out, you need to know that you are working at the correct pace. To do this, you must know what your training heart rate range should be.

There are two parts in determining this:

1. Find your maximum heart rate by subtracting your age from 220.

> e.g: 220 (the given number)
> _____ - 42_ (your age)
> **178   your maximum heart rate**

2. Multiply your maximum heart rate by your workout intensity. This will give you your training heart rate range. Your workout intensity will be maintained between 60% and 85% of your maximum heart rate.

> e.g: 178 (your maximum heart rate)
> _____ x 60%/ 85%_
> 107/151

These figures mean that while you are exercising you should maintain your heart rate between 107 and 151 beats per minute.

220 - _____ (your age) =_____ , your maximum heart rate.

_____ (your minimum heart rate) x 60% =

_____ (your maximum heart rate) x 85% =

Remember these ranges are estimates. There may be times when you will exceed your maximum heart rate. As you become conditioned you may find that you want to do more.

The following chart gives examples of **Work Effort Ranges** for various ages.

WORK EFFORT RANGES

Age (in years)	Range (heart rate)
20	120-170
25	117-166
30	114-162
35	111-157
40	108-153
45	105-149
50	102-145
55	99-140
60	96-136
65	93-132
70	90-128
75	87-123
80	84-119

RESTING HEART RATE

To find this number: Before you get out of bed in the morning, count your heartbeat for 10 seconds and multiply this number by 6. You can also count the number of beats within 60 seconds and use that number as your resting heart rate. We haven't used this number in any of our calculations, but you may see a reference to it in other fitness literature.

THE FOLLOWING ARE FREQUENTLY ASKED FITNESS QUESTIONS, WITH THEIR ANSWERS:

1. How much time will I need to devote to this routine to see changes?
To increase your general fitness level, you can exercise as little as 20-30 minutes a day, three times a week. To lose inches and/or weight, you will need 60 to 90 minutes, four days a week.

2. How will my energy be affected?
You may find your energy level fluctuating during the first one to three weeks of your exercise routine. After that time, you should see an increase in energy.

3. How will my body change?
You will think more clearly, have increased stamina and firmer muscles.

4. Will I be able to oversee and regulate my own exercise program, or do I need to hire a personal trainer?
A personal trainer can help with motivation, as well as watching you for proper breathing, alignment and doing the exercises correctly. But it is, of course, possible to exercise on your own, as you use this book.

5. Will I have to stop eating my favorite foods?
Not necessarily. During the first three weeks of this fitness program, you should follow the four rules for healthy eating. But after that time, you may add other foods you like, in moderation.

6. Will I get sore muscles? Why?
Yes, you probably will. The amount of soreness will depend on how you pace yourself. As you exercise, you are developing new muscle fibers and strengthening old ones. During this process the fibers produce lactic acid and other chemicals that cause pain.

7. Are the rewards of a fitness program worth the effort?
Definitely. Exercising regularly and eating well will improve your life and your attitude. A fitness routine should be a lifetime commitment, a true lifestyle change.

8. *Will I look like the photographs in the muscle magazines?*
   **This is unlikely, unless you have the appropriate genetic makeup.
   But, you will lose fat, gain muscle, improve your appearance and
   feel better about yourself.**

UNDERSTANDING RISK FACTORS

The greater the number of health risk factors you have, the greater
your risk for coronary artery heart disease. The following list
represents some of these factors:

* Hypertension

* Total cholesterol greater than 200 mg./dl

* Cigarette smoking

* LDL cholesterol greater than 130 mg./dl

* HDL cholesterol less than 35 mg./dl

   Age greater than 45 (men)

   Age greater than 55 (women)

* Obesity (30% or more overweight)

* Diabetes Mellitus

   History of stroke or arterial blood clots

Heart attack or sudden death before 55 in a male parent, sibling or
offspring. Heart attack before age 65 in a female parent, sibling,
or offspring.

   **Items with a * are those risk factors which
   can be altered with lifestyle changes,
   such as a change in eating or fitness level.**

OVERCOMING MYTHS

One of the reasons for not staying with an exercise routine is having beliefs that may not be accurate. Some of these are listed below, with accurate information following each one.

Myth: *If I stop exercising, the muscles I have developed will turn to fat.*
Fact: Muscles don't turn to fat. However, fat can develop around and between the muscle fibers.

Myth: *Being overweight will shorten my life.*
Fact: Not necessarily, although obesity has been linked to heart disease, cancer, stroke, hypertension, hyperlipidemia, and gallbladder disease.

Myth: *If I eat too many starchy foods, I will gain weight.*
Fact: False, all foods should be eaten in moderation. Starches, a form of carbohydrate, can supply you with needed energy.

Myth: *I have to eat less than 1000 calories a day to lose weight.*
Fact: False. Any reduction in calories will likely result in eventual loss of some weight. The amount will depend on many factors. Some people have metabolisms that slow down when they cut calories, giving added importance to exercise.

Myth: *To lose fat, I must exercise intensely.*
Fact: False. If you want to lose fat, you must stay within your "Training Heart Rate Range".

Myth: *I won't lose fat if I exercise with weights.*
Fact: False. Weight training, combined with aerobic exercise, will help you lose fat.

Myth: *I am overweight because I have a thyroid problem.*
Fact: This is, of course, possible, but it's unlikely. If you're concerned about this, you should check with your doctor.

Myth: *I am tired all the time so I must have Chronic Fatigue Syndrome.*
Fact: This is also unlikely, although you should check with your doctor if you're concerned. You will be less tired as you follow a regular fitness routine.

Myth: *I have arthritis and exercise will make it worse.*
Fact: Moderate exercise can help with arthritis symptoms.

HOW TO USE THIS BOOK

The most important ingredient you will need is PATIENCE. As you move on in this book, it's important to establish a strong foundation with each chapter. Remember, this requires time and patience. Give yourself both.

As a beginner, it's better to proceed slowly than to go too quickly. You may need to spend as little as one to two weeks doing aerobic exercise (walking/jogging and/or biking) or as much as two to three months before going on to the third chapter. Once you start the third chapter, you may want to spend as long as you think you will need before going on to the next. Even though the days are numbered, if you reach the end of a chapter and want to repeat it, do so before moving on. Purchase a 9 x 6 notebook to write down the answers to the questions that you will be repeatedly answering.

If you are an ambivalent exerciser (someone who has trouble sticking with exercising), you must recognize the reasons you get sidetracked and give yourself an opportunity to overcome them. You may want to consider hiring a trainer, or exercising with a partner as you use the book.

If you are an obsessive exerciser (overly intense), keep your perspective and take time for yourself in ways other than exercise. Pay special attention to the written portion of the workbook and try to learn from your answers.

If you are a balanced exerciser, you have already learned the importance of moderation and the required time and patience to achieve the goals you have or are setting for yourself.

WHAT IS A WORKOUT?

George H. Allen, Chairman of President's Council on
Fitness and Sports (1970-1974) stated that . . .

"A workout is 25% perspiration and 75% determination. Stated
another way, it is one part physical exertion and three parts self-
discipline. Doing it is easy once you get started. A workout makes
you better today than you were yesterday. It strengthens the body,
relaxes the mind, and toughens the spirit. When you work out
regularly, your problems diminish and your confidence grows.

A workout is a personal triumph over laziness and procrastination.
It is the badge of a winner—the mark of an organized goal-oriented
person who has taken charge of his or her destiny. A workout is a wise
use of time and an investment in excellence. It is a way of preparing
for life's challenges and proving to yourself that you have what it
takes to do what is necessary.

A workout is a key that helps unlock the door to opportunity and
success. Hidden within each of us is an extraordinary force. Physical
and mental fitness are the triggers that can release it. A workout is a
form of rebirth. When you finish a good workout, you don't simply
feel better. You will feel better about yourself."

WEIGHT LOSS

If part of your goal is weight loss, it's important to be patient. Losing weight needs to include long term lifestyle modification changes in order to be successful. Unless you undertake a medically supervised, very low calorie program, the best way to lose weight is by losing small amounts over a long period of time.

People who crash diet to lose weight invariably gain all of it back and sometimes more. On the other hand, those who combine permanent improved nutritional intake with a permanent exercise program stand the best long term chance of reaching a goal weight and maintaining that weight.

What about medications for weight loss? Medications should be reserved only for those with significant health risk from being over-weight. When indicated, the addition of medication can further im-prove a person's chances of success.

With *Your Personal Trainer's* overall program an individual can expect long term weight loss, but the pounds may not come off right away. The reason is that initially fat loss is replaced by muscle gain through increased fluid. An individual will lose inches by body mea-surement first. As strength and endurance improve, weight begins to come off. Try not to pay too much attention to the scale in the early stages.

An important part of *Your Personal Trainer* is muscle strengthening exercises. Why is this? Why not just eat right and do aerobic exer-cises? Eating right and aerobic exercises are important, but strength-ening is critical as well. In terms of weight loss, muscle strengthening improves metabolic rate throughout the day. If you decrease your calorie intake alone, eventually almost everyone drops their metabolic rate, making continued long term weight loss less likely. On the average, people who do muscle strengthening will have higher meta-bolic rates one year into a weight loss program than those who do not. The strengthening component of *Your Personal Trainer* in itself does not burn calories at a high rate. Fifteen minutes of strength training burns about 100 calories for a 150 lb. person. However, combined with the aerobic component, it does more to keep your metabolic rate higher than anything else. The higher your metabolic rate, the easier it is to lose weight and maintain that loss long term.

If you tend to have trouble losing weight, avoiding fatty foods will eventually make you lose your desire for their taste. If you are quite overweight and have had a tough time losing weight in the past, you may want to consider counting and limiting fat grams. Individuals who take in 20 grams of fat or less, every day for a year, lose their taste and desire for fat.

With the additional use of medication men can expect 5-10 pounds in the first month and up to 5 pounds thereafter; women can expect 4-8 pounds the first month and 2-6 pounds per month thereafter. Even in the lowest calorie liquid diets consuming only about 600 calories per day, men lose 8-16 pounds per month and women lose 4-8 pounds per month. Therefore, unless you are in a highly medically supervised very low calorie program, do not set your sights too high. Your best bet for continued success is to realize that weight which comes off slowly, if lost in the right way, can be kept off.

CHAPTER ONE

ESTABLISH YOUR FOUNDATION

> **LOOK CLOSELY AT YOURSELF**
> **PAY ATTENTION TO HOW YOU FEEL, THINK AND ACT**
> **MEASURE YOURSELF TO KNOW YOUR STARTING POINT**
> **PLAN A DAILY ROUTINE**
> **BEGIN YOUR EXERCISE ROUTINE**

LOOK CLOSELY AT YOURSELF

Chapter One isn't just the first step of an exercise routine. It's the beginning of a self-examination, mentally, emotionally and physically, that will lead you to a fit and healthy life. This examination begins with fifty questions which will be repeated in the middle and at the end of this book so you can note any changes you have made. Check your response for each question that reflected how you responded to past situations.

1.   *I have lots of energy and I look forward to each day.*
   ☐ Never   ☐ Seldom   ☐ Sometimes   ☐ Often   ☐ Always

2.   *I find a challenge exciting.*
   ☐ Never   ☐ Seldom   ☐ Sometimes   ☐ Often   ☐ Always

3.   *I show good judgment when I experience a difficult situation.*
   ☐ Never   ☐ Seldom   ☐ Sometimes   ☐ Often   ☐ Always

4.   *When I feel rushed and have deadlines to meet, I think of them as challenges.*
   ☐ Never   ☐ Seldom   ☐ Sometimes   ☐ Often   ☐ Always

5.   *I believe that if I persist, I will overcome adversity.*
   ☐ Never   ☐ Seldom   ☐ Sometimes   ☐ Often   ☐ Always

6.   To avoid feeling overwhelmed, I set mental and physical goals
     that are attainable.
     ☐ Never   ☐ Seldom   ☐ Sometimes   ☐ Often   ☐ Always

7.   I believe in my ability to remain faithful to my values.
     ☐ Never   ☐ Seldom   ☐ Sometimes   ☐ Often   ☐ Always

8.   I feel motivated and determined.
     ☐ Never   ☐ Seldom   ☐ Sometimes   ☐ Often   ☐ Always

9.   I can maintain my concentration to achieve a goal.
     ☐ Never   ☐ Seldom   ☐ Sometimes   ☐ Often   ☐ Always

10. To accomplish my goals, I keep myself ready and alert.
     ☐ Never   ☐ Seldom   ☐ Sometimes   ☐ Often   ☐ Always

11. I am happy with the decisions I make.
     ☐ Never   ☐ Seldom   ☐ Sometimes   ☐ Often   ☐ Always

12. When I feel stressed or depressed, I use exercise to relieve
     my feelings.
     ☐ Never   ☐ Seldom   ☐ Sometimes   ☐ Often   ☐ Always

13. When I feel overwhelmed or fatigued, I use a brief period of
     relaxation to rejuvenate myself.
     ☐ Never   ☐ Seldom   ☐ Sometimes   ☐ Often   ☐ Always

14. I eat a balanced intake of food.
     ☐ Never   ☐ Seldom   ☐ Sometimes   ☐ Often   ☐ Always

15.   *I take regular vacations.*
☐Never   ☐Seldom   ☐Sometimes   ☐Often   ☐Always

16.   *I enjoy interacting with others.*
☐Never   ☐Seldom   ☐Sometimes   ☐Often   ☐Always

17.   *I am able to achieve goals I have set for myself.*
☐Never   ☐Seldom   ☐Sometimes   ☐Often   ☐Always

18.   *I have the support I need.*
☐Never   ☐Seldom   ☐Sometimes   ☐Often   ☐Always

19.   *I use incentives to keep me focused on my goals.*
☐Never   ☐Seldom   ☐Sometimes   ☐Often   ☐Always

20.   *When I want to make changes in my life, I ask for help.*
☐Never   ☐Seldom   ☐Sometimes   ☐Often   ☐Always

21.   *I am happy with the choices I have made so far in my life.*
☐Never   ☐Seldom   ☐Sometimes   ☐Often   ☐Always

22.   *I stay motivated so I can accomplish my goals.*
☐Never   ☐Seldom   ☐Sometimes   ☐Often   ☐Always

23.   *I have the incentive, the knowledge and the support to change any unhealthy behaviors.*
☐Never   ☐Seldom   ☐Sometimes   ☐Often   ☐Always

24.   *I act contrary to my common sense and wants.*
☐Never   ☐Seldom   ☐Sometimes   ☐Often   ☐Always

25. *I feel tired for no apparent reason.*
☐ Never   ☐ Seldom   ☐ Sometimes   ☐ Often   ☐ Always

26. *I feel confused and helpless.*
☐ Never   ☐ Seldom   ☐ Sometimes   ☐ Often   ☐ Always

27. *Because I feel uneasy around others, I avoid socializing.*
☐ Never   ☐ Seldom   ☐ Sometimes   ☐ Often   ☐ Always

28. *I have fears which prevent me from acting decisively.*
☐ Never   ☐ Seldom   ☐ Sometimes   ☐ Often   ☐ Always

29. *Other people can make me feel rushed, stressed or worried.*
☐ Never   ☐ Seldom   ☐ Sometimes   ☐ Often   ☐Always

30. *There are times when I don't have the courage to act decisively.*
☐ Never   ☐ Seldom   ☐ Sometimes   ☐ Often   ☐ Always

31. *I feel restless and edgy.*
☐ Never   ☐ Seldom   ☐ Sometimes   ☐ Often   ☐ Always

33. *I have strong fears of situations I'm powerless to control or avoid.*
☐ Never   ☐ Seldom   ☐ Sometimes   ☐ Often   ☐ Always

35. *I feel I've reached a point where I need to make changes, but I'm not motivated.*
☐ Never   ☐ Seldom   ☐ Sometimes   ☐ Often   ☐ Always

36. *I have bowel problems - constipation, diarrhea, pain or bloating.*
    ☐ Never ☐ Seldom ☐ Sometimes ☐ Often ☐ Always

37. *I have brief periods of excessive agitation.*
    ☐ Never ☐ Seldom ☐ Sometimes ☐ Often ☐ Always

38. *I have difficulty functioning as I have in the past.*
    ☐ Never ☐ Seldom ☐ Sometimes ☐ Often ☐ Always

39. *When I feel frustrated with my life, I don't want to face others. I would rather stay home to avoid any contact.*
    ☐ Never ☐ Seldom ☐ Sometimes ☐ Often ☐ Always

40. *I feel depressed.*
    ☐ Never ☐ Seldom ☐ Sometimes ☐ Often ☐ Always

41. *I find myself overeating when I feel stressed or depressed.*
    ☐ Never ☐ Seldom ☐ Sometimes ☐ Often ☐ Always

42. *I have a decreased sex drive.*
    ☐ Never ☐ Seldom ☐ Sometimes ☐ Often ☐ Always

43. *I find it hard to concentrate or feel motivated When I feel like this, I move too slowly to accomplish anything.*
    ☐ Never ☐ Seldom ☐ Sometimes ☐ Often ☐ Always

44. *I have trouble getting the same pleasure from my life I once got.*
    ☐ Never ☐ Seldom ☐ Sometimes ☐ Often ☐ Always

45. *I use alcohol or drugs as a means of relaxation.*
☐ Never ☐ Seldom ☐ Sometimes ☐ Often ☐ Always

46. *I have thoughts of harming myself or committing suicide.*
☐ Never ☐ Seldom ☐ Sometimes ☐ Often ☐ Always

47. *I feel inadequate.*
☐ Never ☐ Seldom ☐ Sometimes ☐ Often ☐ Always

48. *I wish I had taken a different direction earlier in life.*
☐ Never ☐ Seldom ☐ Sometimes ☐ Often ☐ Always

49. *I don't have enough time for myself, my family or my friends.*
☐ Never ☐ Seldom ☐ Sometimes ☐ Often ☐ Always

50. *I have verbal disagreements with others.*
☐ Never ☐ Seldom ☐ Sometimes ☐ Often ☐ Always

LEARN TO PAY ATTENTION

Learning to pay attention to how you feel, think and act will help you understand how negative and positive thoughts and emotions can affect your attitude toward your health and life in general. As you work your way through *Your Personal Trainer*, you will find yourself learning to pay attention not only to how you are feeling physically, but emotionally as well. Learning to recognize and express feelings that affect you negatively and positively will help you change the patterns in your life. Your daily life is a balance of emotional highs and lows. As you understand what produces your range, you can learn to predict or even control some of these feelings. What are the six influences that affect you in your daily life? The following definitions are one way of examining these:

Expectations are essential in anyone's life. But when too much is expected of, you may find yourself feeling pressured. This may lead to a feeling of exhaustion or even depression. Achievable expectations, on the other hand, can make you feel exhilarated and capable.

Everyone has various *roles* they play as part of interacting as a social being. But it's essential that these roles are clearly defined and are personally desirable. If they are vague or too difficult, again you will find your energy level will be decreased. If they are concise and attractive, your life will be enhanced.

Each person is affected by his or her daily *physical environment*. It may be crowded, noisy or polluted in some way. This can make you feel less energetic or even apathetic. A positive environment that is comfortable for you can make you feel enthusiastic and optimistic.

Your *emotional environment* can also control how you feel. If it's hostile, oppressive, confusing or distracting, you can feel discouraged or depressed. But if it's supportive, clear and friendly, it can improve your daily life.

If your *social environment* includes constant disagreements, lack of privacy or feelings of isolation, these can drain your energy. An environment that includes close friends and relaxed relationships can energize and inspire you.

Possibly two of the most important factors to affect your daily energy level is your *perception* of what is happening around you and your **attitude** about the situation. If you are constantly anxious or afraid, you will think and feel exhausted and unmotivated. If you are confident in your ability to handle any circumstance, even difficult ones, you will approach your life with enthusiasm and anticipation.

EXAMINE THE INFLUENCES IN YOUR DAILY LIFE

Throughout *Your Personal Trainer* you'll find exercises in which we have you answer questions and write responses down. It's very important that you physically write your answers, not just think through the responses in your mind. Physical writing solidifies answers in your mind and makes it much easier to draw conclusion and develop solutions.

Just before you go to sleep each night, reflect back over your day. Keep *Your Personal Trainer* near your bed so you can record your thoughts.

How did you feel?

Did you have moments of excitement or anticipation?

Did you have times of lethargy or lack of enthusiasm?

As you recall the moments, answer these questions:

1. Did one or more of the six influences affect you today because of circumstances in your recent or distant past?
e.g.: I've been having feelings of loneliness, fear of failure, and uncertainty about my future.

2. Did one or more of these influences affect you today because of present circumstances?
e.g.: I don't get along with my co-workers or supervisor and so I am tense and tired at work.

4. *List the actions you took today to relieve yourself of the results of one of these influences.*
e.g.: I find the drive to work exhausting and frustrating, so I took public transportation today.

5. *List one or more of these influences that made you feel enthusiastic and excited today.*
e.g.: I had lunch with an old friend whom I haven't seen in a long time. I'd forgotten how much I like her and she likes me.

Read back over these questions and your answers.
Do you have any thoughts on what you've written?

As a result of this self-examination, you will gradually find yourself able to understand how your daily activities and attitudes affect your motivation. You will find that setting goals, both physical and emotional, and being persistent in achieving them, will become easier. *Your Personal Trainer* will provide you with the structure for acting on your physical and emotional goals. It will also continue to encourage examination of the emotional decisions you make every day. It is the interaction of these decisions and this structure that will allow you to make changes in your daily lifestyle and your physical well-being.

TAKE YOUR MEASUREMENTS

The previous questions looked at your present emotional attitudes, so that you will be able to see how they change, as you progress in this routine. This section provides the same for your physical self. Using either a soft tape measure or a string, take each of these measurements and write them on the chart.

BODY PART	MEAS. DATE	GOAL DATE	FOLLOW-UP DATE	FOLLOW-UP DATE
Neck	_____	_____	_____	_____
Shoulder	_____	_____	_____	_____
Chest	_____	_____	_____	_____
Breast	_____	_____	_____	_____
Abdomen	_____	_____	_____	_____
Waist	_____	_____	_____	_____
Hips	_____	_____	_____	_____
Right thigh	_____	_____	_____	_____
Right calf	_____	_____	_____	_____
Left thigh	_____	_____	_____	_____
Left calf	_____	_____	_____	_____
Right arm	_____	_____	_____	_____
Right forearm	_____	_____	_____	_____
Left arm	_____	_____	_____	_____
Left forearm	_____	_____	_____	_____

My weight today is _____

My goal weight is _____   Follow up goal weight is _____

For exact locations of each measurement, see diagram on next page.

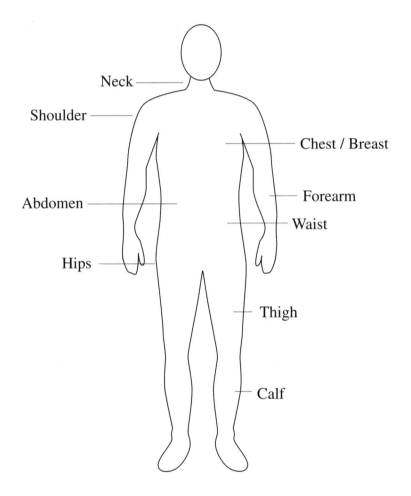

PLAN A DAILY ROUTINE

Take a moment and think back to a favorite trip you've taken. Think about the anticipation and planning that went into it. There were decisions to be made about your destination and the duration of your trip. You may have been anxious about whether you could afford it or take the time from your work life. But you know you need to take the time for yourself and so you move from the fantasy of taking the trip to the reality. You decide where to go, how long you will stay, and what you will do while you're away.

You can look at your daily life in the same way. Instead of being anxious about what each day's routine will look like, you can plan your daily goals. For each day you can:

- Decide your daily destinations

- Identify possible outcomes

- Prepare for contingencies

- Set up your daily schedule

- Make careful choices

- Follow through

If you look at your daily life as a trip you're planning, you can feel more in control and meet each day with enthusiasm. The anticipation of meeting your chosen goals can affect your attitude toward all of your life. For example, when you're going on a trip, you may find yourself less bothered by daily stresses that normally would make you anxious or concerned. Because you have your trip to look forward to, you have a different perspective. Setting goals that include exciting and rewarding results can give you the same perspective in your daily life.

Examples of goals you may have for yourself are:

- Making new friends
- Getting more pleasure from life

- Challenging yourself
- Relaxation

Setting and accomplishing goals is an important step in feeling optimistic about your life. Structuring your daily time will help you with this. The time exercises in *Your Personal Trainer* will allow you to consciously eliminate daily activities that slow you down and increase activities that help you accomplish your goals. You will learn new habits that will allow you to approach your life feeling optimistic and in control.

REALISTIC EXPECTATIONS

Begin with realistic expectations. How much weight do you think is a reasonable goal to lose each week or each month? Many people vastly overestimate the rate at which pounds should come off, leading to early frustration and, as a result, breakdown in motivation. A reasonable goal for weight loss from improved nutritional intake, exercise and behavioral changes is 2-4 pounds per month for men and 1-2 pounds per month for women. These values may look small, but remember this does not involve crash dieting or drastic calorie reduction, but instead a reasonable goal that an individual can achieve and maintain. This rate means losing 24-48 pounds per year for men and 12-24 pounds per year for women.

KEEPING TRACK OF YOUR TIME

Your first week gives you an idea of how you are spending time. In each daily task you are to enter the time in which you accomplish the task. You will be writing the times of your daily tasks only once this week. However, make sure you make mental notes of all these tasks daily so you can compare them. You can also choose which day to keep track of these tasks. Whichever day you chose make sure you complete the whole day.

DAILY ROUTINE

1. What time did you wake up?
2. What time did you get out of bed?
3. How long did it take you to eat breakfast?
4. What time did you leave for work/school/other?
5. What time did you arrive at work?
6. What time did you start work?
7. How long did it take you to eat your first snack?
8. What were your work hours after you finished your snack?
9. How long were your break times?
10. How long did it take you to eat your lunch?
11. What were your working hours after you finished your lunch?
12. How long did it take you to eat your second snack?
13. What time did you leave work?
14. What time did you get home?
15. What time did you have your dinner meal?
16. When did you watch television?
17. How much time did you take for personal quiet time?
18. When will you exercise?
19. How much time did you devote to family time?
20. How much time did you devote to work study?
21. How much time did you devote to pleasure reading?
22. How much time did you devote to school study?
23. How much time did you devote to socializing with friends?
24. How much time did you devote to chores?
25. What time did you go to bed?

DAY 1   TODAY'S DATE:
WALKING OR BIKING

One of the most effective workouts for all body types is walking, followed by a series of stretches. It's gentle, easy to avoid injury and will give you a sense of accomplishment during the beginning stages of your routine. Another excellent way to begin an exercise routine is with biking. Using an exer-cycle at home or at a gym will give you control over the time of day and the level of exercise you do. If you have already been walking for exercise, you may have already chosen a route. If not, there are two important factors to consider when you walk outside. First, the terrain should be flat so you can have a consistent pace. Second, to avoid breathing in carbon monoxide, choose an area with as few cars as possible. If you are a member of a health club, you can use the treadmill there for walking. Both the walking and the biking are for time and not distance. Because you will need some way of keeping track of the time, and also be able to check your pulse, use a watch with a second hand.

FOR THOSE ALREADY ON AN EXERCISE PROGRAM

Do you already routinely do an established exercise routine such as jogging, stepping, rowing, swimming, etc.? If so, you may substitute that exercise for biking or walking. Exercise for 30 minutes. Take a full water bottle with you, so you can sip water as you exercise. This will keep your body internally cool and replace what you lose during exercising.

AVOIDING INJURY—PROPER SHOES

To avoid injury, it's critical to wear the proper shoes. First, buy shoes that are designed for your activity. They should have a firm sole to provide support. Soft-soled shoes can feel good when you first put them on, but as you exercise, your feet will tire quickly. If you have a high arch, you may need to use a firm arch support to prevent overuse injuries, such as shin splints. Be cautious when buying an air support shoe. For some people air soled shoes do not provide good support and can more easily lead to injury.

Answer the following questions before you get started:
How do you feel before starting your workout? (Check one or more)

☐ Motivated   ☐ Discouraged

☐ Excited   ☐ Dreading

☐ Pressed for time ☐ Resigned

☐ Confident   ☐ Anxious

☐ Not sure   ☐ Ready and willing

☐ Clear-minded   ☐ Don't want to think about it

Do you know why you're doing this?   *Yes   No   Explain:*

WALK/JOG OR BIKE FOR HEALTH

Starting time:____ Starting heart rate:____ Goal heart rate: From____to____

The first six minutes of your walk are important. During this time, your bones and muscles will be adjusting to your walking surface. Bend your arms at the elbow and swing them with a slight twist at the waist. Make the length of your stride comfortable.

> *At five minutes thirty seconds, slow your stride so you can check your heart rate. At 6 minutes, the time is_____ and my heart rate is_____. Resume your pace.*

You should now be approaching your training zone heart rate. If you have already reached this target rate, slow down. As you continue, notice how you feel. You will be writing about this later. During the next six minutes, your body temperature will begin to rise and you will start to utilize carbohydrates for energy.

> *At 11 minutes 30 seconds, slow your pace and check your heart rate. At 12 minutes the time is____and my heart rate is_____.*

You should now be in the middle of your training zone. If your heart rate is below this number, increase your speed. If you are above it, slow your pace. You should now be feeling hot and you may be perspiring. Your breathing will be faster because your body is asking for more oxygen. Take deep, controlled breaths.

It's usually at this point that you will find yourself thinking of other activities you could be doing. Or you may find yourself wanting to push harder, so that your heart rate is out of the training zone. Both of these are common reactions to exercise. It's important to keep going at the correct pace, neither slowing down or pushing yourself too hard.

> *At 17 minutes 30 seconds slow your pace and check your heart rate.*
> *At 18 minutes the time is_____ and my heart rate is_____.*

You should still be in the middle of your target range. If you are, maintain your current pace. Otherwise, speed up or slow down as needed. Your target range is the ideal heart rate for cardiovascular exercise, as well as metabolizing carbohydrates and fats. If you are above this range, you will metabolize less.

> *At 23 minutes 30 seconds slow down and check your heart rate.*
> *At 24 minutes the time is_____ and my heart rate is _____.*
>
> *You will now begin to slow your pace and begin your six minutes of cooling down. At 30 minutes the time is _____ and my heart rate is _____.*

STATIONARY BIKING FOR HEALTH

Before you start your bicycling, you should have the bicycle seat at the correct height. Adjust it so that the seat is even with your hipbone when you are standing next to it. Record this setting:_____

Starting time____Starting heart rate____Goal heart rate: from___to___

Sit upright and begin pedaling slowly. The first six minutes of your ride gives your body and mind a chance to adjust to the exercise. At five minutes thirty seconds, slow down, if necessary, and begin to take your pulse.

At 6 minutes, the time is____ and my heart rate is_____.
Resume your pace.

You should now be approaching your training zone heart rate. If you have already reached this target rate, slow down. As you continue, notice how you feel. You will be writing about this later. During the next six minutes, your body temperature will begin to rise and you will start to utilize carbohydrates for energy.

At 11 minutes 30 seconds, slow down if necessary, and check your heart rate. At 12 minutes the time is____and my heart rate is _____.
Resume your pace.

You should now be in the middle of your training zone. If your heart rate is below this number, increase your speed. If you are above it, slow your pace. You should now be feeling hot and you may be perspiring. Your breathing will be faster because your body is asking for more oxygen. Take deep, controlled breaths.

It's usually at this point that you will find yourself thinking of other activities you could be doing. Or you may find you want to push yourself harder, so that your heart rate is out of the training zone. Both of these are common reactions to exercise. It's important to keep going at the correct pace, neither slowing down or pushing yourself too hard.

At 17 minutes 30 seconds slow your pace, if necessary, and check your heart rate. At 18 minutes the time is _____ and my heart rate is _____.

You should still be in the middle of your target range. If you are, maintain your current pace. Otherwise, slow down or speed up as needed. Your target range is the ideal heart rate for cardiovascular exercise, as well as metabolizing carbohydrates and fats. If you are above this range, you will metabolize less.

> *At 23 minutes 30 seconds slow down, if necessary, and check your heart rate. At 24 minutes the time is _____ and my heart rate is_____*

> *You will now begin to slow your pace and begin your 6 minutes of cooling down. At 30 minutes the time is _____ and my heart rate is _____*

Follow-up Questions - ask yourself these questions.

How did you feel while you were exercising?
(Check one or more answers)

☐ Needed more energy   ☐ Distracted by negative thoughts

☐ Could have gone on forever   ☐ My body really hurt

☐ Energetic   ☐ Powerful

☐ Active   ☐ Enjoyment

☐ Fun   ☐ Invigorated

Did you feel self-motivated?   *If not, why not?*
If you did, what was motivating you?

How did you feel after you exercised? (Check one or more)

☐ Glad it's over   ☐ Joyful

☐ Can't wait until next time   ☐ Poised

☐ Dreading next time   ☐ Gratified

☐ I wish I had started this long ago ☐ Renewed

☐ Now I understand why this is important ☐ Rejuvenated

☐ Feel good about what I accomplished ☐ Successful

This exercise made me feel I am on my way to becoming more fit.

Yes   No   Explain:

It's important to finish your workout by stretching your body. Your stretching is done right after your cardiovascular workout. (Chapter 9, pgs. 1 -12) Hold your stretch for 20 seconds.

DAY 2   TODAY'S DATE:
NO EXERCISE

Today there will be no physical routine, but instead there will be written exercises. Day 2 provides an opportunity to gain insight into how you respond to the occurrences in your life. Do you expect too much of yourself? Do you respond tensely to demands from others? Is your behavior predictable? These are questions for you to consider and answer.

This book does not contain recipes or an extensive diet plan. Instead, we encourage you to combine a healthy nutritional intake with continued exercise. You will find yourself making better food choices as you begin to feel more fit. The purpose and the belief behind this book is the importance of making a lifestyle commitment, not just a temporary one.

BLOOD PRESSURE & HEALTH

Have you had your blood pressure checked recently? Do you under-stand what the top and bottom numbers mean in a blood pressure reading?

Very simply, the top number (systolic) is the pressure in the arteries while the heart is making each contraction. The bottom number (diastolic) is the pressure while the heart is resting in each cycle. Of the two numbers, the bottom number was previously considered the most important in controlling hypertension (HTN), because the heart is at rest twice as long as it is contracting. However, recent data indicates that the systolic blood pressure is as important to control as the diastolic pressure. Did you know that the heart beats an average of 100,000 times a day?

Can you imagine doing that many repetitions of any muscle work? A crucial part of good health is assuring yourself that your blood pressure is normal. Normal is generally considered to be less than 130/85, at rest. Borderline HTN is 130-140/85-90 and true HTN is 140/90 or greater. Increased blood pressure puts excessive wear and tear on the arteries leading to the heart and brain. Over years this wear and tear blocks the arteries and can lead to heart attacks and strokes. Thus, control of blood pressure is crucial to health and longevity. If your blood pressure is too high, what can you do to control it on your own? Hypertension can be self-controlled in various people to varying degrees. An excessive salt intake can have a significant adverse effect on blood pressure.

Many foods, such as chips, mayonnaise, ketchup, mustard, cheese, soda, various fast foods, bottled or canned salad dressings, etc., have hidden salts. Limiting these foods can significantly drop the blood pressure in some people. Exercise will often decrease blood pressure as well. However, in many people, blood pressure may only decrease by as little as five points. Some people will see a larger drop when long term exercise is achieved. If your blood pressure doesn't drop much after months of work, don't be discouraged.

There are many reasons for exercise and many benefits besides the effect on blood pressure. Exercising will dramatically decrease your risk of heart attack and stroke, even if it doesn't drop your blood pressure much. If your blood pressure reading is above 140 systolic or 90 diastolic, consult your physician, as further treatment (usually with medication) is critical to your long term health.

DAY 3   TODAY'S DATE:
WALKING OR BIKING

Varying your routine, by alternating bicycling and walking, is a good idea. These exercises use muscles differently and you will find the variety more interesting. So if you walked on Day 1, and if you have access to a bicycle or exer-cycle, follow the biking routine today. If not, continue walking. Either way, follow the same time and heart rate schedule. Use this chart to keep track of both. Be aware of how you feel before, during and after your workout. Remember the written exercise you did on Day 1. It is a good idea to do the same today.

WALK/JOG		OR	BIKE	
Time _____	*HR* _____		*Time* _____	*HR* _____
*Start*_____			*Start*_____	
@ 6 min	_____		@ 6 min	_____
@12 min	_____		@ 12 min	_____
@18 min	_____		@ 18 min	_____
@24 min	_____		@ 24 min	_____
@30 min	_____		@ 30 min	_____
Stop _____			*Stop* _____	

After you finish this workout, follow your cardiomuscular flexibility routine. Hold each stretch for 20 seconds. Whenever you stretch, make sure you count to 20 for each body part.

STRESS & ANXIETY—IS STRESS NORMAL?

Some degree of stress and anxiety are a part of everyone's life. A small amount of stress can actually be beneficial, helping you to be more efficient, avoid boredom and reach some of our goals. Exercise has a large effect on stress. A person with no stress in their life may be bored and need more stimulation. Exercise can often be an excellent first step toward a heightened energy level and toward increased self-motivation.

In an overly stressed person, exercise can provide a way of releasing stress, as well as providing an outlet. It can create a feeling of optimism and well-being. But for people who are highly stressed, exercise alone may not be adequate. When stress reaches the point that it feels uncontrollable, there may be various physical manifestations. These can include an inability to sleep or concentrate, a lack of energy and motivation, and fast-moving thoughts which will not stop. There may also be headaches, neck aches, body aches and upset stomach, including diarrhea. If symptoms like these appear, a physician should be consulted. Counseling and medication may need to be added to your exercise routine.

It's important not to exercise vigorously close to bedtime. Although it may refresh your mind, your body may feel like being up and around and you may not be able to sleep. On the other hand, if you're feeling sleepy during the day and you need to be alert, that's a great time to exercise. Forty-five minutes after exercising, most people feel refreshed and ready to go.

Now, go back over your time schedule to see where there might be potential problems. Where do you need more time? Less time? Start asking yourself questions about your daily time schedule. The rest of the week you will be asked to do the same mental exercise. Try to concentrate on improving how you manage your time.

Tonight, put *Your Personal Trainer* by your bedside, and allow a few extra minutes in the morning for written exercises before you get out of bed.

DAY 4
A DAY OFF

TODAY'S DATE:

Today is a day off from physical exercise. Instead you will be doing a written exercise and continuing a healthy intake of food. On Day 2 you had an opportunity to look closely at your responses to daily occurrences. The six influences that affect you each day were listed and discussed. As you examined them, you were encouraged to look back over your day and think of how you felt and behaved. You then suggested ways you could take more control over your daily life. Take a moment to think back over the six influences and their definitions.

As you complete these new written exercises, you will start to examine how your unconscious hours of sleep are affecting you during the day and how your awareness of this can lead to positive changes in your daily feelings and behaviors.

Answer these questions before you get out of bed this morning:
How did you feel when you woke up?

Did you get enough sleep? If not, why not?

If you dreamed, how did your dreams make you feel about yourself?

If a dream affected you negatively, what do you need to work on today to help you think more positively about yourself?

Answer these questions before you leave home:
How do you feel as you leave for school or work?

Do you feel motivated and clear about what you want to accomplish today? If not, what can you do to change this?

Answer these questions when you return home today:
How did you feel during your day?

Did you plan all your activities for the day?　　*Yes　or　No*
Were you able to stay with these plans?　　*Yes　or　No*

If no, what happened?

What could you do next time to prevent this from happening?

Answer these questions at the end of your day:
How do you feel as your day is ending?

Did you accomplish what you wanted to accomplish? Explain.

If you did, how can you reward yourself?

If you weren't able to reach your goals, what steps can you take to help you come closer tomorrow?

Repetition of behaviors and thoughts has an ongoing impact on your life. If you want to change some of your old habits and develop new ones, it's essential that you set clear goals and stay with them. Whatever thoughts or actions you repeat over and over will become the thoughts or actions that you have habitually. Answering these questions daily will allow you to become aware of your present habits and change them if you want them to be different. You will find you have control in areas you may have thought uncontrollable. Tomorrow you will be walking or biking. Take a few minutes now to think about exercising: Why are you exercising? How are you feeling about it? Imagine yourself as an exercising person, one whose habit is exercise and good nutrition.

WHAT HAPPENS DURING EXERCISE?

Whenever you perform normal exercise, microscopic damage is done to muscles so that the exercise can occur. This damage occurs to the micro filaments in the muscle tissue as the muscle contracts and expands to create work. The harder the force of contraction (e.g., weight lifting and aerobic exercise), the more damage is done. Muscle damage is not to be confused with more serious and less easily healed damage of an injury such as a sprain or strain. Normal recuperation of muscles following exercise takes forty-eight hours. This allows actin and myosin filaments to heal and rebuild so more exercise can be undertaken. For this reason, a particularly strenuous exercise (e.g., weight lifting for an isolated body part) isn't recommended two days in a row.

Your Personal Trainer will be instructing a variety of exercises. For example, lower body parts one day and upper the next. You will also alternate intense aerobic activities, jogging or bicycling, and have periodic days of complete rest to allow full muscle recovery. If muscles aren't allowed a recovery phase, performance and energy levels drop off and the risk of injury increases dramatically. As you age, this fact becomes even more important. Remember that you will need to allow forty-eight hours for muscle recovery.

You might wonder why a high performance athlete, such as a marathon runner, is able to run every day. These athletes can exercise at a lower level without doing any damage, just as you may take a stroll without doing damage. A low level exercise day can still allow healing. So, a high intensity athlete can alternate hard and light exercise days or even two hard days alternating with one light one. The light day acts as a recovery day, even though the athlete is still exercising that day.

To alternate muscles exercised you can alternate your activities on various days. For example, you might jog Monday, Wednesday and Friday, but bicycle or swim on the alternate days.

DAY 5   TODAY'S DATE:
WALKING OR BIKING

Today you will concentrate on increasing your workout time.
Follow the same routine as on Day 1.

WALK/JOG	OR	BIKE
Time _____ *HR* _____	*Time* _____	*HR* _____
*Start*_____	*Start*_____	
@ 6 min _____	@ 6 min	_____
@12 min _____	@ 12 min	_____
@18 min _____	@ 18 min	_____
@24 min _____	@ 24 min	_____
@30 min _____	@ 30 min	_____
@36 min _____	@ 36 min	_____
Stop _____	*Stop* _____	

SIGNS OF DEPRESSION

Are you experiencing any of the following symptoms? Difficulty
concentrating? Chronic headache? Sleep problems? A problem using
your time efficiently? Constant fatigue? Too much tension? Any or all
of these may be symptoms of an underlying depression. We tend to
think of depression as a feeling of being constantly tearful and sad, as
is the case with acute depression. However, chronic or chemical
depression may be much more subtle. Seventy percent of patients
report sleep troubles, loss of or increased appetite, weakness, fatigue,
headaches, or agitation as the primary symptoms of depression.

National statistics show that six percent of the United States population will experience a major depression episode sometime in their
lifetime. Ten to twenty percent of patients seeing a family doctor will
report one or more of the symptoms that indicate an underlying
depression.

What criteria are diagnostic of chemical depression?
A diagnosis of major depression can be made if a depressed mood and/
or decreased interest in daily activities lasts more than two weeks,
and there are at least four of the following symptoms:

- significant appetite or weight change
- change in sleep pattern: insomnia or hypersomnia
- fatigue or loss of energy
- poor concentration or indecision
- suicidal thoughts or recurrent thoughts of death
- feelings of worthlessness or inappropriate guilt

Depression can sometimes be so subtle as to cause only nonspecific
complaints, such as pain, fatigue and dizziness, or some symptoms of
other diseases. It can disrupt a person's capacity to work and maintain
social and familial relationships. Expense can become an issue, as
patients often undergo extensive medical workup before depression is
diagnosed. The most serious consequence of depression is suicide.
It is estimated that more than half of the patients who commit suicide
have visited a doctor within the preceding month, often with vague
complaints other than "I'm depressed."

Treatment of Depression - Major depression is a confirmed medical
illness that seems to be caused by a chemical imbalance in the brain,
not just a form of personal maladjustment. The treatment varies with
the severity. Sometimes simply waiting will allow it to resolve on its
own. Exercise can be beneficial, as it stimulates the body and the
mind. Counseling may be helpful and, in some cases, antidepressant
medication may be required. If you have any of the signs or symptoms
of depression discussed here, you may want to seek the advice of a
doctor.

What's Normal? - If you've read the above information on depression
and found yourself saying, "Yes, I feel a little sad at times, but that's
all," then you are experiencing a normal part of life. Give yourself a
little kick by eating a healthy food intake and by getting the adrenaline
pumping with a good exercise program, such as this one. Keep at it
and in most cases that blue, unmotivated feeling will lift.

DAY 6   TODAY'S DATE:
MEDITATION: A TIME FOR SILENCE

Your Personal Trainer lists two types of meditation routines.
One concentrates on engaging you physically and the other on
maintaining quietness of mind. Practice both and alternate them.

A time for silence will help you clear your mind of thoughts that may
be interfering with your life. For example, you may have been in
situations when you needed to quiet the voice inside your head.
Because of this negative voice, you weren't able to enjoy yourself.
To begin this process start by giving yourself fifteen minutes and
follow these steps:

MEDITATION I

1 Choose a quiet place where you won't be disturbed.

2 Sit in a comfortable position, feet flat on the floor,
   and close your eyes.

3 Concentrate your attention only on your breathing. Become aware
   of the soft sensations of your breath as the air flows in and out
   through your nose.

4 As thoughts and images come into your mind, let them come and
   go without examining them.

5 Instead of trying to control your breathing, just be aware of it.
   It may speed up or slow down, but concentrate only on the full
   exhalation and inhalation and the pauses in between.

6 Your goal is to reach a state of awareness without being distracted
   by particular thoughts or feelings.

7 If you find your mind wandering, bring your focus back to your
   breathing. When you first start this exercise, you will probably
   find this happening frequently. But with daily practice it will get
   easier and easier.

8 Have patience with yourself. The benefits of silence are subtle but
   important. Use this time to clear your mind of any negative or
   critical thoughts.

MEDITATION II

Find a quiet spot away from people. Read the following instruction first:

1 Close your eyes and think through this process.

2 Start by focusing on your toes and work your focus gradually up your body. As you progress, spend ten to fifteen seconds focusing on each body part. Spend longer if you can.

3 After focusing on your toes, focus on your feet, then your ankles, your knees, etc. up to your lungs, your heart, then to your neck, head, eyes and scalp.

4 While focusing on each area direct a part of your attention to your breathing. Take slow deep breaths in and out. Feel yourself inhaling and exhaling. Picture breathing in something very positive such as the warmth of a good friendship or the feeling you have for a loved one.

5 As you breathe out, picture pushing out negative feelings such as frustration or anger.

6 Breathe in the positive and breathe out the negative, as you continue to focus on each part of your body as well.

7 When you reach the uppermost part of your head or scalp, picture yourself opening up to a whole new positive world. Then gradually bring yourself back to an awareness of the world around you.

8 Now that you've read through the above meditation, go ahead and close your eyes and spend fifteen minutes doing the exercise.

9 Each time you do this exercise, you'll find you get something more out of it. If you have any trouble remembering it all, you might close your eyes and have someone lead you through it once or twice. You can also tape record yourself reading these instructions.

FLUIDS & DEHYDRATION

As you follow this program stay aware of your fluid intake. The current recommendation for fluids by the American College of Sports Medicine is a pint of water fifteen to thirty minutes before exercising. Cold fluids are preferable to warm fluids since they pass through the stomach more rapidly. For every pound lost during exercise, a pint of fluid is lost. For the exercises in this book, hydration with cool water alone is fine for fluid replacement.

However, if you are performing high endurance sports, it is helpful to hydrate with fluids that also contain sodium and carbohydrates. Adding carbohydrates in the form of a glucose polymer or glucose-fructose solution helps stop glycogen depletion, delays muscle fatigue and prolongs endurance. Many brand names of carbohydrate sodium solutions are now available. If you are performing an endurance event you should drink 100 to 300 ml every 20-30 minutes during the event. If you are running more than 2 hours (e.g. marathon), drink a carbohydrate beverage that contains 6 to 8 percent carbohydrate concentration. Check the bottle for carbohydrate concentration and type of carbohydrate. The beverage should contain fructose, glucose, sucrose, maltodextrine, glucose polymer or some combination of these.

Long distance runners can lose up to 6 liters of fluid during a run and dehydration can decrease an athlete's performance.

DAY 7   TODAY'S DATE:
WALKING AND BIKING / COMBINING ROUTINES

On Day 1 you either chose a walking/jogging route or started to use an exer-cycle. On Day 3, you changed to walking/jogging or biking, so you could use your muscles differently. Day 5 saw an increase in time with either of these forms of exercise. Today, Day 7, you will do twenty minutes of walking and 20 minutes of biking for a forty minute cardioendurance workout. If you do not have a bike, then walk for the full forty minutes.

Be aware of how you feel before during and after your work out.

W A L K, J O G	**AND**	**B I K E**
Time _____ HR _____		*Time _____ HR _____*
Start_____		*Start _____*
@ 6 min _____		@ 6 min _____
@ 12 min _____		@ 12 min _____
@ 18 min _____		@ 18 min _____
@ 24 min _____		@ 24 min _____
@ 30 min _____		@ 30 min _____
Stop_____		*Stop _____*

It's important to finish your workout with stretching of your body. Hold each body part stretch for a 20 second count.

CHAPTER TWO

STRENGTHEN YOUR FOUNDATION

ESTABLISH YOUR GOALS
CHOOSE AN EXERCISE FACILITY
EXAMINE YOUR EATING HABITS
CONTINUE YOUR EXERCISE

DAY 8   TODAY'S DATE:
INCREASING YOUR EFFORT

Before you start your exercise today, be aware of how you feel before starting your workout. By understanding your attitude toward exercising, you will be able to challenge yourself to work harder. If you are dreading your workout, it will be difficult to sustain this or any lifestyle change routine that incorporates exercise as a motivating energy. Therefore it's essential for you to understand your thoughts and help yourself develop new, more positive ones related to productive lifestyle change.

> *It's important to choose a course or exercise facility where you feel comfortable or you may not look forward to exercising.*

WORKOUT: WALKING OR BIKING

Before you start your workout, enter your start time and your beginning heart rate. Check your heart rate every six minutes. To keep track of these numbers, you can either keep your notebook with you as you exercise, or remember to record them later. Today you will be working out for thirty minutes. Take your water bottle with you, so you can sip water as you exercise.

WALK/JOG		OR	BIKE	
Time _____ *HR* _____			*Time* _____ *HR* _____	
Start _____			*Start* _____	
@ 6 min	_____		@ 6 min	_____
@12 min	_____		@ 12 min	_____
@18 min	_____		@ 18 min	_____
@24 min	_____		@ 24 min	_____
@30 min	_____		@ 30 min	_____
*Stop*_____			*Stop* _____	

FLEXIBILITY STRETCHES

Now that you have finished your walk, jog or bike ride, it's time for your flexibility stretches. These exercises are important because they condition your muscles and allow them to adjust as you exercise. When you have finished stretching, you will have completed your exercise for today. Stretches are located in chapter 9, pages 1 -12.

EXERCISE & WEIGHT LOSS

The role exercise plays in losing weight is more than simply the calories burned during your workout. If you workout at more than fifty percent capacity, you will INCREASE your metabolic rate for as long as twenty-four hours. The calorie usage will increase all day and night, including the time you are not exercising. Also when you do aerobic exercise, your appetite for high calorie foods will be suppressed.

A common question asked about the metabolic rate is, "Why am I not losing weight? I'm eating less and I'm exercising more." If you exercise and eat less you would expect to lose weight. However, in the first 4-6 weeks, often weight does not change much. Let's take the following example to explain why:

> A woman weighs 150 lbs and eats 1800 calories to sustain her 150 lb weight. She has a body fat of 25%. She exercises using our program and burns 225 calories per day. Her metabolic rate increases for the 24 hours by an additional 75 calories per day. She is actually burning 300 calories more per exercise day. Her appetite drops, so she now eats only 1500 calories per day. So, she now burns 2100 calories per day but eats only 1500 calories. After one month she still weighs 150 pounds. She is frustrated. Should she be? What happened? Six hundred calories less per day should cause her to lose about a pound of fat per week or 4 pounds per month. Therefore, she actually burned four pounds of fat during the month and her body fat is now down to 22.5%. However, she added 4 pounds of combined muscle (i.e. protein) weight and water weight. She still weighs the same amount but she is much more fit. As the months go by, she will continue to burn fat but won't need to build more muscle so she will start to lose weight.

CALORIES & DIGESTION

Whenever you eat food, calories are used to digest food. This is called the "thermic effect" of food. High protein foods have the highest thermic effect, while carbohydrates have a lower thermic effect. The thermic effect may double following exercise, so if you exercise and then eat, it takes more calories to digest the food you've eaten.

DAY 9   TODAY'S DATE:
EXAMINING YOUR EATING HABITS

Examining your eating habits will make the difference between success and failure. Why, where and when you eat is just as important as what you eat. Today there will be no workout. Instead, you will continue to examine your eating habits and learn more about your daily calorie needs. To provide the proper fuel for your body, you must eat a healthy balance of fats, proteins and carbohydrates. This balance will help you maintain your energy level throughout the day. The easiest way to control your nutritional intake is to bring foods from home rather than eating out. This will not only provide you with healthy food, but will give you a chance to learn about the right foods for you. Continue to keep a written record of the foods you are eating, how you feel as you eat them, and why, where and when you eat.

Answer these questions today:
What are you thinking about and how do you feel before you eat?

Breakfast

Snack I

Lunch

Snack II

Dinner

Snack III

What are you thinking about and how do you feel as you are eating?
Each time you eat, think about why, where and when you are eating.

Breakfast

Snack I

Lunch

Snack II

Dinner

Snack III

What are you thinking about and how do you feel after you've eaten?

Breakfast

Snack I

Lunch

Snack II

Dinner

Snack III

DAILY CALORIC REQUIREMENTS & EXERCISE

These are affected by the intensity and duration of your exercise. The amount of calories needed is also controlled by the outside temperature, your body's surface area, your age and your sex. A highly skilled athlete (i.e. professional swimmer) may need as many as five thousand calories a day, while a sedentary person may need only twelve to fifteen hundred. It's important to know your approximate calorie needs. Staying within this range will help you control your weight and maintain your energy level.

CALORIE REQUIREMENTS ARE A COMBINATION OF:

Basal Energy Rate + daily activity needs + energy expended during exercise.

You can calculate your approximate basal energy rate (also called Basal Metabolic Rate or BMR) by using the following formula:

For women: 10 -11 x weight in pounds
For men: 11-12 x weight in pounds

Now add your daily activity needs as follows:

30% of your BMR if you perform light work (such as desk job, household tasks, light industrial)

50% of your BMR if you perform moderate work (construction, factory work)

100% of your BMR if you perform strenuous work (forest workers, miners)

Now add your energy expended during exercise using the chart on the next page.

> ***Listed in the table below are approximate calories expended per hour by weight.***

Example calculation: A 150 lb female executive does a brisk walk daily. Her approximate calorie requirements are:
BMR + Daily activity need + energy expended during exercise = calories (10x150) + (.3x1500) + 198 = 1500 + 450 + 198 = 2148 calories to maintain body weight. Of course if she was trying to lose weight, her calorie intake will need to be less.

Body Weight	*200–180*	*170–150*	*140–120*	*110–100*
Weight Lifting	444	426	378	330
Running (11 min. mile)	714	630	552	480
Biking (10mph)	474	438	372	324
Aerobic Dancing	516	468	396	340
Swimming (slow crawl)	805	720	636	552
Basketball (half court)	636	564	486	268
Basketball (full court)	870	792	396	348
Calisthenics	474	438	270	234
Jogging (5 mph)	762	690	588	516
Golf (walking)	468	390	348	300
Dancing	558	474	420	366
Lawn Moving	312	288	240	210
Sex	348	318	270	234
Gardening	657	516	456	396
Cleaning	396	270	252	222
Cooking	330	210	186	162
Tennis	696	630	534	468

continued >

Body Weight	200–180	170–150	140–120	110–100
Stair climbing	528	474	402	354
Skiing (downhill)	798	738	624	468
Skiing (cross country)	1158	1056	888	786
Skating (vigorous)	720	654	558	486
Biking (stat. 10 mph)	492	444	378	330
Biking (stat. 20 mph)	1032	936	798	702
Walking (2 mph)	216	198	168	144
Walking (4 mph)	408	366	312	270

The calories you expend during a physical activity depend not only on the activity, but on your weight and how hard you are working. Use the information above to get a general idea of how many calories you may be burning per one hour. Find your activity and choose the weight range closest to your weight.

PROPER NUTRITION

. . . is important for all athletes, from beginners to professionals. Eating the right foods improves your performance, as well as helping you maintain a sense of well-being and self-esteem.

DAY 10   TODAY'S DATE:
WALKING OR BIKING

Today is another day of either walking, jogging or biking. You may find you enjoy alternating these activities. If you are going outside to walk, either take a small notebook with you or remember your heart rates and record them when you return home. You will be walking for thirty minutes or biking for twenty-four. Check your heart rate every six minutes. Don't forget to take your water bottle with you, so you can sip water as you exercise. Make a mental note of the following:

- *How do you feel before starting your workout?*
- *Do you know why you're doing this?*
- *How do these answers compare to your previous ones?*
- *Is there a difference?   Why?*

WALK/JOG		**OR**	**BIKE**	
Time _____ *HR* _____			*Time* _____ *HR* _____	
Start _____			*Start* _____	
@ 6 min	____		@ 6 min	____
@12 min	____		@ 12 min	____
@18 min	____		@ 18 min	____
@24 min	____		@ 24 min	____
@30 min	____		@ 30 min	____
Stop _____			*Stop* _____	

Make a mental note of these questions:

- *How did you feel during your workout?*
- *Were you able to keep yourself motivated?*
- *How do you feel now that your workout is finished?*

STRETCHES

Now that you have finished your walk or bike ride, it's time for your flexibility stretches. Hold each body part stretch for 25 seconds.

EATING DISORDERS

Bulimia and anorexia nervosa are two eating disorders.
Some of the symptoms of bulimia include:

A. Very strict dieting

B. Vigorous over-exercising to prevent weight gain

C. A persistent and excessive concern with body shape and weight

D. Recurrent episodes of binge eating, with a minimum of two binge episodes a week for at least three months

E. Lack of control over binge behaviors

F. Regularly inducing vomiting or using laxatives or diuretics.
Anorexia nervosa includes A, B and C above, as well as:

G. An intense fear of gaining weight

H. A disturbed body image
(thinking you are fat no matter how little you weigh)

I. Lack of *or* irregular menses in women

Women are ten times as likely to have an eating disorder as men.
The typical woman with this problem is single, college educated,
Caucasian and middle to upper class. Other groups of affected women
are flight attendants, fashion models and athletes. Bulimia and
anorexia men include athletes (particularly jockeys), figure skaters,
gymnasts, body builders, wrestlers, divers, swimmers and distance
runners. Bulimia is ten times more common than anorexia for both
men and women. The more severe forms of anorexia and bulimia
carry a ten percent chance of death. If you think you may have an
eating disorder, it's best to consult with a physician.

***It's important, as you work your way through this, to stay
aware of the influences that affect you in your daily life.
So again, take the time tonight just before you go to sleep
to write out . . .***

How are your past experiences affecting you now?

How are your present experiences affecting you now?

Are you achieving your present goals?

*What actions did you take today to rid yourself of any negative
influences?*

*What influences did you experience today that made you feel
enthusiastic and excited?*

*Read back over these questions and your answers.
Do you have any thoughts on what you've written?*

*Read back over these questions and your answers.
Do you notice any patterns?*

Answer these questions before you get out of bed in the morning:
How did you feel when you woke up?

Did you get enough sleep? If not, why not?

If you dreamed, how did your dreams make you feel about yourself?

If a dream affected you negatively, what do you need to work on today to help you think more positively about yourself?

Answer these questions before you leave home:
How do you feel as you leave for school or work?

Do you feel motivated and clear about what you want to accomplish today? If not, what can you do to change this?

Answer these questions when you return home:
How did you feel during your day?

Did you plan all your activities for the day? Yes   or   No   If no, what happened?

Were you able to stay with these plans?   Yes   or   No   If no, what happened?

What could you do next time to prevent this from happening?

Answer these questions at the end of your day:
How do you feel as your day is ending?

Did you accomplish what you wanted to accomplish? Explain.

If you did, how can you reward yourself?

If you weren't able to reach your goals, what steps could you take to help yourself come closer tomorrow?

Repetition of behaviors and thoughts has an ongoing impact on your life. If you want to change some of your old habits and develop new ones, it's essential you set clear goals and stay with them. Whatever thoughts or actions you repeat over and over will become the thoughts or actions you have habitually.

Knowing your daily task routine will help you in the process of taking control of your daily life and the tasks that you perform each day.

DAILY ROUTINE

1. What time did you wake up?

2. What time did you get out of bed?

3. How long did it take you to eat your first meal?

4. What time did you leave for work/school/other?

5. What time did you arrive at work?

6. What time did you start work?

7. How long did it take you to eat your first snack?

8. What were your working times after you finished your snack?

9. How long were your break times?

10. How long did it take you to eat your lunch?

11. What were your working times after you finished your lunch?

12. How long did it take you to eat your second snack?

13. What time did you leave work?

14. What time did you get home?

15. What time did you have dinner?

16. When did you watch television?

17. How much time did you take for personal quiet time?

18. When did you exercise?

19. How much time did you devote to family time?

20. How much time did you devote to work / study?

SMOKING

We all know smoking is harmful, but just how harmful? We can estimate that for every one minute a person smokes, his or her life span is reduced by about an average of one minute. Smoking increases the risk of coronary disease, stroke and many cancers, including a few lung, throat and mouth cancers. How does one stop smoking?
The first step is to raise your motivation, set a stop date and, to resist any temptation, throw away any left over cigarettes.

Instead of smoking, substitute something else for oral gratification, such as chewing gum, carrot sticks or a straw. If you've tried to quit in the past and have gone back to smoking, try again. People who try to quit over and over again eventually make it. There may be some initial side effects: irritability, increased appetite, or anxiety. In time these symptoms will subside.

There are many aids to help people quit smoking. Some use fear of cancer or dying, by reflecting on a loved one or friend. Others use peer pressure or an awareness of just what they are doing when they smoke. Teenagers respond best to the non-glamorous appearance of smoking, both to quit and prevent them from starting. In some people, additional supportive therapy works, such as biofeedback, hypnosis, behavioral modification and counseling.

Some people are helped by nicotine containing medications, such as the patch, on a temporary basis. This approach allows you to break the psychological addiction of having a cigarette in one's hand at first, and then later to break the physical addiction to nicotine. There are various patches available. There is also nicotine gum, as well as nicotine nasal spray, and soon an inhaled nicotine will be available. If you are a smoker, keep trying various approaches, until you find the one that works for you. It can be done.

DAY 11   TODAY'S DATE:
MEDITATION: A TIME FOR SILENCE

Today is a day off from physical exercise, but you should continue to eat well. One way to help you become aware of the way your body and mind is affected by the thoughts and stresses of daily life is to give yourself a mental respite. So, again, take some time to work on silencing your thoughts. As before, take fifteen minutes for this exercise. Choose meditation I or II.

*Tomorrow will be another opportunity
to continue your goal of exercise and good health.*

DAY 12   TODAY'S DATE:
WORKOUT: WALKING/JOGGING OR BIKING

Before you start your workout, enter your start time and your beginning heart rate. To keep track of these numbers, you can either keep your notebook with you as you exercise, or remember to record them later.

How do you feel before starting your workout?

Do you know why you're doing this? Yes   No   Explain:

How do these answers compare to your previous ones?

If there is a difference, why?

W A L K / J O G   OR   B I K E

Time _____ *HR* _____   *Time* _____   *HR* _____
Start _____   *Start* _____
@ 6 min   _____   @   6 min   _____
@ 12 min   _____   @ 12 min   _____
@ 18 min   _____   @ 18 min   _____
@ 24 min   _____   @ 24 min   _____
@ 30 min   _____   @ 30 min   _____
Stop _____   *Stop* _____

How did you feel during your workout?

Were you able to keep yourself motivated?
If so, how? If not, why not?

How do you feel now that your workout is finished?

STRETCHES

It's now time for your flexibility stretches.
Hold each body part stretch for 25 seconds.

MENOPAUSE, ESTROGEN AND EXERCISE FOR WOMEN

Women can help prevent two major causes of morbidity (injury and illness) and mortality (death) after menopause by doing exercise and taking *postmenopausal estrogen.* There is now clear cut evidence that both aerobic exercise and postmenopausal estrogen significantly reduce the risk of coronary artery disease in wormen.

The effect of estrogen may be great enough to negate elevated cholesterol. *Osteoporosis* (and subsequent hip fractures in elderly women) is a far too common cause of major disability and often eventual death. The addition of estrogen starting at menopause, along with weight bearing exercise throughout life, play a major role in reducing the risk of osteoporosis. Estrogen has some drawbacks as well, but should be discussed at length with a woman's physician as menopause approaches.

DAY 13   TODAY'S DATE:
A DAY OFF

Today, instead of exercising, you will learn more about physical fitness.

MUSCLE CRAMPS

What causes muscle cramps? No one knows exactly what causes them, but there are many factors that contribute to them. Some people seem to be predisposed to cramps and may need to be more careful than others. If you suffer from frequent muscle cramps, you may want to consider some of the contributing factors and see if they apply to you.

- Electrolyte imbalance from dehydration may be the cause. Make sure you are drinking plenty of fluids.

- Cramps seem to be more common in early summer before people get acclimated to the warmer weather.

- Dieters who exercise are particularly susceptible to cramps because of inadequate sodium, potassium, calcium and magnesium intake. Being sure to include these in your food may help alleviate cramps.

- Cold weather, muscle fatigue, inadequate training and sudden increase in activity may all contribute to muscle cramps.

- People who are just beginning or returning to exercise may experience cramping if they overwork. A gradual approach to training can be helpful.

- Frequent, recurring cramps can be a sign of serious underlying disease, including neurologic disease, vascular disease or diabetes. However, millions of people suffer from occasional cramps without having any serious disorder.

There are two kinds of muscle cramps. *Night cramps* occur at rest after exercise and usually involve the calf and foot muscles. *Heat cramps* occur during or shortly after exercise and usually they affect the hands and large leg and arm muscles. These are the cramps caused by electrolyte imbalance and dehydration. Heat cramps can be the first sign of heat stroke.

There are many treatments available for cramps. Simply stretching the muscle is probably the most effective. Massage is helpful by increasing blood flow to get rid of metabolic waste. Ice also increases the blood flow and numbs the muscle. Fluid replacement is important and can be achieved by using an electrolyte solution.

BALANCING YOUR LIFESTYLE

The most important message we want to give you about your life is the idea of balance or equilibrium. There will be many influences in your daily life. Some of these will be positive and some negative. These influences may work against each other, and you will find yourself out of equilibrium. In order for you to understand the results of this
imbalance, it's important to stay aware of how you feel each day. Our questions about outside influences help you conduct an accurate self-evaluation of your daily experiences. As you continue in this book and even after you've finished, your observations about the influences in your life will help you feel more in control of your life. Negative experiences may not be preventable, but your reactions to them can be changed.

DAY 14   TODAY'S DATE:
WALKING/JOGGING AND BIKING

Over the past thirteen days, you have conducted a progression of physical and mental exercises. *Your Personal Trainer* has assisted you in becoming aware of combining these exercises, so you can make changes within your life. Chapter One emphasized establishing your foundation by taking an emotional inventory, learning to pay attention to how you think and feel, measuring your body, planning a daily routine and beginning to exercise.

On Day 1 you either walked/jogged or bicycled, drank plenty of water and checked your pulse periodically, to determine your training zone. There was also an emphasis on becoming aware of how you think about your physical effort before, during and after you exercise. Day 1 ended with stretching to loosen you up and help your blood flow.

On Day 2 you took the day off from your physical routine to concentrate on your written exercises and on understanding the importance of proper food intake. On your next exercise day, Day 3, you were assigned to do alternating exercise, so your muscles could adjust to new demands. On Day 4 you took another day off, but you concentrated on understanding how unconscious hours of sleep can affect your waking hours. Day 5 saw an increase in your exercise time.
On Day 6 you took another day off from physical exercise but started a meditation routine to have time for quiet. On Day 7, you did twenty minutes of biking and twenty minutes of walking for increased endurance.

On Day 8 you started putting more effort into your workout. You also continued to examine how you think and feel before, during and after you exercise. The day ended with stretching (cardiomuscular flexibility) to loosen you up and help your blood flow. On Day 9, you took the day off from your physical routine to concentrate on your written exercises related to what you think about before, during and after you eat. Your next exercise day, Day 10, you either did walking/jogging or biking and at the end of your aerobic work, you finished the routine with stretching.

On Day 11 you took another day off and, with meditation, concentrated on becoming aware of the way your body and mind are affected by the thoughts and stresses of daily life. Day 12 saw an increase in your exercise time followed by your stretch routine. On Day 13 you took another day off from physical exercise. In today's routine, Day 14, you will perform both walking/jogging and biking to increase your endurance. If you do not have a bike, walk/jog for the hour.

Think about these questions before you start.
How do you feel before starting your workout?

Do you know why you're doing this? Yes   No   Explain:

How do these answers compare to your previous ones?
If there is a difference, why?

W A L K / J O G   A N D   B I K E

Time _____ *HR* _____   *Time* _____ *HR* _____
*Start*_____   *Start*_____

@ 6 min _____   @ 6 min _____
@ 12 min _____   @ 12 min _____
@ 18 min _____   @ 18 min _____
@ 24 min _____   @ 24 min _____
@ 30 min _____   @ 30 min _____
*Stop*_____   *Stop* _____

How did you feel during your workout?

Were you able to keep yourself motivated? If so, how? If not, why not?

How do you feel now that your workout is finished?

STRETCHES

It's again time for your flexibility stretches. Hold each body part stretch for 25 seconds. As you finish Chapter Two, take a few minutes to look back at your daily time schedules. Are you satisfied with how you are using your time? If you are, you're taking control of your life.

TIME GOALS:
What are six ways you created time for yourself during this chapter?

1._____ 2._____

3._____ 4._____

5._____ 6._____

What are six more goals you have which could create even more time for yourself?

1._____ 2._____

3._____ 4._____

5._____ 6._____

OVEREATING - HAVE WE FOUND A CAUSE?

For years medicines for weight loss were considered taboo by the medical profession. However, since the early to mid 1990's, doctors' understanding and approach to weight loss has fluctuated rapidly.

Doctors now believe that individuals who overeat and are overweight often do so because of a chemical imbalance in the brain. It's not completely because of some emotional problem or stress that some people overeat, but instead because they may lack needed chemicals in certain parts of the brain. Doctors know that serotonin centers exist in the brain, and if serotonin is low, individuals have a decreased satiety that tells them to eat. Most likely norepinephrine and tryptophan and a number of other hormones also play roles.

Many health care professionals now consider obesity to be a disease. Obesity increases the risk of coronary artery *disease, stroke, diabetes, fatty liver disease, hypertension, cholesterol problems, gallbladder disease, arthritis and cancer of the colon, rectum and breast.* As a result, medications have been advocated to attempt to decrease an individual's weight and thereby decrease health risk. Unfortunately, with widespread use of these medications, health risks such as pulmonary hypertension and valvular heart disease have been reported, and some medications have been removed from the market for further study.

Consult your health care professional for the latest developments. Also remember that medication is for those overweight enough to have significant health risk from their weight, not for slightly overweight individuals. Medicine has rarely been effective alone, but must be combined with proper nutritional intake, aerobic and strengthening exercises and an effective behavioral modification program. Again the key to long-term success is long-term behavioral change.

> *If you've reached this point and feel that you'll need more time just walking/jogging and/or biking, continue to do this. In Chapter Three you'll begin to perform resistance exercises. If you think you need to continue to walk/jog and/or bike for the next two or three months it won't distract you from your weight training effort. If you choose to do this, we recommend you purchase a three subject notebook, 9 1/2 inches by 6 inches. This will allow you to continue your daily writing.*

CHAPTER THREE

CHALLENGE YOURSELF

> **ASSESS WHAT YOU HAVE LEARNED**
>
> **DEFINE YOUR NEXT GOALS**
>
> **UNDERSTAND THE FUNDAMENTALS OF EXERCISING**
>
> **BEGIN TO TEST YOUR PERSEVERANCE**

DAY 15   TODAY'S DATE:
ASSESS WHAT YOU HAVE LEARNED

There is a natural resistance to continuing any difficult activity, whether emotional or physical. Sometimes stopping or changing the activity is the appropriate response. But there are times when persistence can lead to a sense of accomplishment and increased confidence. So, while it's important to know when to stop, it's equally important to be willing to work beyond some discomfort, slowly and carefully, to see just how far you are capable of going without hurting yourself.

TIME GOALS

At the end of Chapter Two you looked again at the goals you had set for yourself. How were you able to make time for these goals? List the ways here:

You also listed the goals you weren't able to meet. Explain here why you think you weren't able to meet these:

What is the difference between your first and second set of goals? Sometimes a goal can be hard to achieve because it's unrealistic. If you think that's true for some of your goals, take the time now to re-examine them. Discard any that are unrealistic.

DEFINE YOUR NEXT GOALS:

As you progress through this chapter , work on previous goals. At the same time, choose three of your realistic, unaccomplished goals and work toward them. Today you will be comparing your goal times to your actual times. Before you start, sit down and enter in all of your goal times. At the end of the day compare your goal times with your actual times. How do they compare?

DAILY ROUTINE

1. What time do you want to wake up?

   Goal_____   Actual _____

2. What time do you want to get out of bed?

   Goal_____   Actual _____

3. How long will it take you to eat your first meal?

   Goal_____   Actual _____

4. What time will you leave for work/school/other?

   Goal_____   Actual _____

5. What time will you arrive at work?

   Goal_____   Actual _____

6. What time will you start work?

   Goal_____   Actual _____

7. How long will it take you to eat your first snack?

   Goal_____   Actual _____

8. What will be your working times after you finish your snack?

   Goal_____   Actual _____

9. How long will your break be?

   Goal_____   Actual _____

10. How long will it take you to eat your lunch?

Goal_____   Actual _____

11. What will be your working times after you finish your lunch?

Goal_____   Actual _____

12. How long will it take you to eat your second snack?

Goal_____   Actual _____

13. What time will you leave work?

Goal_____   Actual _____

14. How long will it take you to get home?

Goal_____   Actual _____

15. What time will you have your second meal?

Goal_____   Actual _____

16. How much time will you spend watching television?

Goal_____   Actual _____

17. How much time will you take for personal quiet time?

Goal_____   Actual _____

18. How much time will you devote to exercise?

Goal_____   Actual _____

19. How much time will you devote to family time?

Goal_____   Actual _____

20. How much time will you devote to work / study?

Goal_____   Actual _____

21. How much time will you devote to pleasure reading?

Goal_____   Actual _____

22. How much time will you devote to school / study?

Goal_____   ___   Actual _____

23. How much time will you devote to socializing with friends?

Goal_____   ___   Actual _____

24. How much time will you devote to chores?

Goal_____   ___   Actual _____

25. What time will you go to bed?

Goal_____   ___   Actual _____

Setting and accomplishing goals is an important step in feeling optimistic about your life. Structuring your daily time will help you with this.

UNDERSTAND THE FUNDAMENTALS OF EXERCISING

There are five aspects to exercise:
Type, Duration, Intensity, Frequency and Mode.

■ Type—refers to the kind of exercises you are performing. With this program you will be doing combinations of cardiovascular training (aerobic) walking, jogging, rowing, stepping and bicycling, resistance training (anaerobic), calisthenics and weight lifting. There are others types of cardiovascular training that you may be doing now or want to do, for example, swimming, hiking, roller blading, tennis, running, outdoor biking, etc.

■ **Duration**—is the amount of time spent exercising in one session. During these sessions the time will vary from forty-five minutes to one hour and a half.

■ **Intensity**—is the amount and level of your exercise. In Chapter Three, this will be between 60 and 75 percent of maximum heart rate(mhr) and as you progress in the book your rate, in some cases, will reach up to 85–90 % of your mhr.

■**Frequency**—is how often you exercise. Your sessions will vary between three and six times per week.

■ **Mode**—is the structure of your exercise. Your training sessions will provide you with a circuit training approach, which incorporates aerobic (cardiovascular) and anaerobic (resistance) training plus stretching. This mode of exercise allows you to receive the maximum benefits in the least amount of time.

AEROBIC EQUIPMENT

While you can walk or use stairs to exercise aerobically, here is a list of other equipment you may choose to have at home:

Stationary or Airdyne bicycle	Aerobic Steps
Nordic Track Skier	Treadmill
Rower	Power Board

RESISTANCE EQUIPMENT:

If you decide to use weights for resistance training, you will be using all of the equipment listed below:

> ***Three, five and ten pound dumbbell weights***
> for strength training

If you want to develop size, as well as strength, you will also need to have
> ***twenty, thirty, forty, fifty and sixty pound dumbbells.***
It's best to buy the adjustable bar and add the weight plates yourself, so you can add or subtract weight as you wish.

- ■ *Twenty pound adjustable ankle weights*
- ■ *An adjustable flat bench*
- ■ *A set of barbells, and a pulley machine*
  (an assortment of benches is ideal)

While you are working out, remember to:

- Focus on the part of the body you are exercising

- Visualize each movement before you perform it

- Imagine what your body will look like because you are exercising

- Stay aware of the changes you are making

- Control your exercise so you don't work too hard or too little

To avoid injury while using weights, it's important to execute each movement correctly. For overall fitness and health, the number of repetitions is more important than the amount of weight you are using. So don't sacrifice good form for extra weights. Be honest with yourself about your progress. Learn to assess where you are and give yourself the time you need to go farther. The goal is lifetime fitness.

THE DUAL APPROACH

Beginning now, you will combine your cardiovascular workout with muscular endurance exercises. These will vary so you will be using your whole body in a variety of ways. During this time you will be elevating your heart rate to its training zone and maintaining it there while doing resistance exercises. As you exercise, you may find yourself wanting to stop before you are finished. Persevere. The ability to continue will give you greater fitness and also a sense of accomplishment that will extend to other parts of your life.

Cardiovascular is defined by the level of your heart rate and the amount of time you engage in an aerobic effort. Weight resistance is defined by the number of sets, reps and the amount of pounds you lift. *Your Personal Trainer* has developed these modes of exercises:

1. Cardiomuscular Preparation

2. Cardiomuscular Endurance

3. Cardiomuscular Intensity

For your cardiovascular exercise, you will be either biking, walking/jogging or rowing. Before you begin, look at the chart below and find your work effort ranges.

WORK EFFORT RANGES

Age (in years)	Range (heart rate)
20	120–170
25	117–166
30	114–162
35	111–157
40	108–153
45	105–149
50	102–145
55	99–140
60	96–136
65	93–132
70	90–128
75	87–123
80	84–119

OPPOSING MUSCLE GROUPS

The next group of exercises will alternate opposing muscles groups, such as biceps and triceps or quadriceps and hamstrings. Because your legs are the largest group of muscles in your body and therefore require more energy, we will begin with them.

ABOUT PAIN

It's important to trust your own decisions about how much discomfort you can tolerate as you exercise. Everyone has a different exercise history, as well as pain threshold, and so it's impossible to give exact numbers for each person. If you are new to exercising, you may find many of these routines uncomfortable, as well as awkward. This is normal. But you must judge how much discomfort you can or want to tolerate. Be alert for pain that may be a sign of more than sore muscles. It's best to proceed cautiously, especially in the beginning. As you become accustomed to the exercises, you will be better able to decide how much you can ask of your body.

ASPIRIN

Aspirin can be taken for prevention of heart attacks, strokes and cancer. Aspirin taken daily acts as a blood thinner. Platelets are a key factor in the blood, and aspirin thins the blood by making platelets less sticky. Aspirin prevents a clot from forming in the blood vessels that supply blood to the heart muscle and to the brain.

To some degree, with time, plaque builds up in coronary (heart) vessels and cerebral (brain) vessels in almost everyone. A piece of this plaque may tear off or open up in a vessel and the body naturally tries to fix the tear by forming a clot. However, this clot can fully block the coronary vessels or cerebral vessels causing an acute heart attack or stroke. If a person has been taking aspirin, the aspirin can prevent the clot from forming thereby preventing the heart attack or stroke and even saving a person's life.

As one reaches an age at which a stroke or heart attack becomes more likely, based on risk factors, it may be life saving to take aspirin. Only small doses of aspirin are necessary to prevent heart attacks or strokes. One baby aspirin daily or one aspirin every other day is usually sufficient. More is usually not better, due to potential side effects. Consult your physician to determine the age at which your risk may be enough to warrant taking aspirin and the does that would be best. Note that aspirin is contranindicated in certain patients, especially those with a history of gastrointestinal bleeding and those taking coumadin.

Coumadin is another type of blood thinner and mixing with aspirin will thin the blood too much. Aspirin also works as an antioxidant and may be helpful in preventing certain cancers.

WORKOUT: CARDIOMUSCULAR PREPARATION

In Chapter Three you will begin your cardiomuscular preparation workouts. These workouts allow you to begin to prepare your body and mind for the physical and mental challenges you will encounter, as well as testing your ability to persevere.

HOME OR GYM WORKOUT: LOWER BODY ROUTINE

How do you feel before starting your workout?

☐ Motivated   ☐ Discouraged   ☐ Excited

☐ Dreading   ☐ Pressed for time   ☐ Resigned

☐ Anxious   ☐ Confident   ☐ Ready and willing

☐ Not sure   ☐ Clear-minded   ☐ Don't want to think about it

Do you know why you're doing this?   Yes   No
Explain:

How do these answers compare to your previous ones?

Is there a difference?

Why?

> *Keep track of your heart rate as you exercise. Compare your target heart rate to your actual rate, so you can stay aware of how hard you are working. Check your heart rate every 6 minutes and record it, quickly comparing the numbers as you go.*

W A L K / J O G   OR   B I K E

Time _____ *HR* _____   *Time* _____   *HR* _____
Start _____   *Start* _____
@ 6 min   _____   @   6 min   _____
@ 12 min   _____   @ 12 min   _____
@ 18 min   _____   @ 18 min   _____
@ 20 min   _____   @ 20 min   _____
Stop _____   *Stop* _____

Rest for sixty seconds before starting the next part of this workout.

LOWER BODY ROUTINE—CHAPTER 9, PAGES 13 - 25

1. Standing Alternating Leg Curls - 1 set of 12 reps
Smaller builds use 6 - 20 lb weights
Larger builds use 10 - 40 lb weights
After you finish this exercise, do a 20 second count for your hamstring stretch then proceed immediately to:

2. Seated Leg Extension - 1 set of 12 reps
Smaller builds use 10 - 40 lb weights
Larger builds use 20 - 60 lb weights
If you have had knee injuries or if you experience any discomfort using weights for this exercise, do the leg movements without weights and tighten your muscles on each rep. This action will help you develop strength. Finish with a 20 second count quadriceps stretch then proceed immediately to:

3. Standing Leg Adductor (inner thighs)—1 set of 12 reps
Smaller builds use 4 - 40 lb weights
Larger builds use 10 - 60 lb weights
Finish with a 20 second count stretch for your inner thigh muscles then proceed immediately to:

4. Standing One Leg Calf Raises—*1 set of 15 reps - no weights*
Finish with a 20 second stretch for each calf muscle then proceed to
Mid Section Routine: Chapter 9, pages 26 - 29

5. Flat Back Leg Raises—*1 set of 25 reps with no added weight*
Proceed immediately to:

6. Flat Back Crunch Ups— *set of 25 reps*
Proceed immediately to:

7. Side Crunches—*1 set of 25 reps for each oblique.*
Proceed immediately to:

8. Flat Stomach Back Raises—*1 set of 25 reps*

How did you feel while you were exercising?

☐ Needed more energy   ☐ Distracted by negative thoughts

☐ Could have gone on forever   ☐ My body really hurt

☐ Energetic   ☐ Powerful

☐ Active   ☐ Enjoyment

☐ Fun   ☐ Invigorated

Were you able to keep yourself motivated? If so, how? If not, why not?

How do you feel now that your workout is finished?

☐ Glad it's over   ☐ Joyful

☐ Feel good about what I accomplished   ☐ Poised

☐ Can't wait until next time   ☐ Gratified

☐ Dreading next time   ☐ Renewed

☐ I wish I had started this long ago   ☐ Rejuvenated

☐ Now I understand why this is important ☐ Successful

I think and feel I am on my way to becoming more fit.
    Yes   No   Explain:

Trainer's Comments & Suggestions:

EXAMINING THE AFFECTS OF
THE SIX INFLUENCES IN YOUR DAILY LIFE

Just before you go to sleep tonight, reflect back over your day. How did you feel? Did you have moments of excitement or anticipation? Did you have times of lethargy or lack of enthusiasm? As you recall these moments, write your response:

How are your past experiences affecting you now . . .
(positively, negatively?)

How are your present experineces affecting you now . . .
(positively, negatively?)

Are you achieving your present goals?

What actions did you take today to rid yourself of the results of any negative influences?

What actions did you experience today that made you feel enthusiastic and excited?

Read back over these questions and your answers.
Do you have any thoughts on what you've written?

DAY 16 TODAY'S DATE:
WORKOUT: CARDIOMUSCULAR PREPARATION

Before you start your resistance training, you'll be warming up. Since you are exercising your upper body today, it's best that you start your routine with the rower. However, if you don't have one, you can walk or bike. If you have a machine with which you can do upper and lower movement,, use that. It will help you warm up your upper body muscles as well.

WALK/JOG		OR	ROW	
Time _____ *HR* _____			*Time* _____ *HR* _____	
*Start*_____			*Start* _____	
@ 6 min	_____		@ 6 min	_____
@12 min	_____		@ 12 min	_____
@18 min	_____		@ 18 min	_____
@20 min	_____		@ 20 min	_____
Stop _____			*Stop* _____	

UPPER BODY ROUTINE—CHAPTER 9, PAGES 30 - 40

1. Bent Over Rows—1 set of 12 reps
Smaller builds use 12- 40 lbs
Larger builds use 30 - 80 lbs
If you experience pain in your lower back or have lower back problems, you may not want to do this exercise until you first consult with your doctor. Finish with a 20 second count stretch for the back muscles then proceed immediately to:

2. Push-ups or Chest Press—1 set of 12 reps
Smaller builds use 30 lbs
Larger builds use 100 lbs
Finish with a 20 second count stretch for the chest muscles then proceed immediately to:

Make sure you are drinking plenty of water.

3. Overhead Lateral Pulls —1 set of 12 reps
Smaller builds use 8 – 10 lbs
Larger builds use 25 lbs
Finish with a 20 second count stretch them proceed immediately to:

4. Flat Bench Flies —1 set of 12 reps
Smaller builds use 8-10 lbs
Larger builds use 25 lbs
Check your heart rate: Target____   Actual____
Finish with a 20 second count stretch for the chest muscles then proceed immediately to:

5.   Lateral Deltoid Raises —1 set of 12 reps
Smaller builds use 5 lbs
Larger builds use 20 lbs
Finish with a 20 second count stretch for your deltoids and then proceed immediately to:

6. Tricep Kick Backs —1 set of 12 reps
Smaller builds use 6 lbs - Larger builds use 15 lbs
Finish with a 15 second count stretch for the tricep muscles then proceed immediately to:

7. Concentrated Bicep Curls—1 set of 12 reps
Smaller builds use 10 lbs
Larger builds use 25 lbs
Finish with a 20 second count stretch for your bicep muscles then proceed immediately to:

8. Flat Back Leg RAises —1 set of 25 reps
Proceed immediately to:

9. Flat Back Crunch Ups — 1 set of 25 reps
Proceed immediately to:

10. Side Crunches —1 set of 25 reps for each oblique.
Proceed immediately to:

11. Flat Stomach Back Raises—1 set of 25 reps

Now that you have finished this workout, be aware of:

How you felt during your workout

How you were able to keep yourself motivated

Why you were able to persevere

How you feel now that your workout is finished

Do you think and feel you're on your way to becoming more fit

Trainers Comments & Suggestions:

DAY 17   TODAY'S DATE:
MASSAGE

The seventeenth day is the ideal time to have your first massage. Taking the time to have a massage is one of the best gifts you can give yourself. A massage reduces tension as well as any muscle soreness you may be experiencing from your new exercise routine. One of the most important benefits of massage is learning the feeling of relaxation. An experienced masseuse or masseur will find the sore and tense areas in your body and work with you so you can learn to recognize the soreness and tension as it happens. With repeated massages, you will begin to notice the difference between a tense body and a relaxed one. This is an important step because it is part of the self-awareness you will need to maintain a healthy body. Exercise, making informed decisions about your eating and learning to recognize the difference between a tense body and a relaxed one: These are all essential. Without them, any changes you make will be temporary. Taking the time and spending the money to have a massage is an investment in your ongoing well-being.

FOLATE FOR WOMEN

All women of childbearing age should add folate to their nutritional intake. This is not for exercise, but instead to help prevent spinal chord (neural tube) defects in the fetus, should they become pregnant. Defects occur at the time of conception and since over half of the babies born in the U.S. are conceived unexpectedly, women should take folate regularly. The dose is 0.4 mg./day for women in the reproductive years and 1 mg/daily in women with a history of previous pregnancies with neural tube defects.

Folate is also mportant in prevention of heart attack in people who have excessive *homocystine (an amino acid)* in their blood. Folate helps metabolize and get rid of excessive homocystine. All adults should take 0.4 mg. as part of a daily vitamin regimen.

DAY 18   TODAY'S DATE:
CARDIOMUSCULAR PREPARATION
Lower Body Routine

Before getting started, reflect on the following questions:

How do you feel before starting your workout?

Do you know why you're doing this?

How do these answers compare to your previous ones?

Is there a difference? Why?

     W A L K / J O G   **OR**   **B I K E**

WALK/JOG		BIKE	
*Time*_____ *H Rate*_____		*Time* _____ *H Rate*_____	
*Start*_____		*Start* _____	
@ 6 min	_____	@ 6 min	_____
@12 min	_____	@ 12 min	_____
@18 min	_____	@ 18 min	_____
@20 min	_____	@ 20 min	_____
Stop _____		*Stop*_____	

Rest for 60 seconds before beginning the next exercises.

Follow the lower body routine for Day 15, pages 9 -12.

Now that you have finished this workout, be aware of:

How you felt during your workout

How you were able to keep yourself motivated

Why you were able to persevere

How you feel now that your workout is finished

Do you think and feel you're on your way to becoming more fit

Trainers Comments & Suggestions:

DAY 19   TODAY'S DATE:
WORKOUTE: CARDIOMUSCULAR PREPARATION
UPPER BODY ROUTINE

Before getting started, reflect on the following questions:

How do you feel before starting your workout?

Do you know why you're doing this?

How do these answers compare to your previous ones?

Is there a difference?   Why?

R O W

*Time*_____ *Heart Rate*_____
*Start*_____
@ 6 min　　　_____
@12 min　　　_____
@18 min　　　_____
@20 min　　　_____
Stop _____

W A L K / B I K E

*Time*_____ *Heart Rate*_____
Start _____
@ 6 min　　　_____
@ 12 min　　　_____
@ 18 min　　　_____
@ 20 min　　　_____
*Stop*_____

Rest for 60 seconds before beginning the next exercises.

Follow the upper body routine for Day 16, pages 14-15.

Make sure you are aware of:

　　How you felt during your workout

　　How you were able to keep yourself motivated

　　Why you were able to persevere

　　How you feel now that your workout is finished

　　Do you think and feel you're on your way to becoming more fit

Sometime during the day, answer these questions before or after each meal:

What are you thinking about and how do you feel before you eat?

　　Breakfast

　　Snack I

　　Lunch

　　Snack II

　　Dinner

　　Snack III

What are you thinking about and how do you feel as you are eating?

Breakfast

Snack I

Lunch

Snack II

Dinner

Snack III

What are you thinking about and how do you feel after you've eaten?

Breakfast

Snack I

Lunch

Snack II

Dinner

Snack III

Do you see any link between your emotions and your eating patterns? Some people eat because they're upset, frustrated, angry, etc. If you find this happening, remember you can learn to replace overeating or unhealthy eating with healthier choices.

DAY 20   TODAY'S DATE:
MEDITATION: A TIME FOR SILENCE

Today is a day off from exercise. Instead, choose meditation I or II for 20 minutes. Meditation is another way to help you become aware of the way your mind and body are affected by the thoughts and stresses of daily life. This time is an opportunity to take a break from your life routine. As you quiet your mind and focus only on the moment, you will find yourself relaxing. When you return to your life and your usual thoughts, you will be refreshed and invigorated. So, again, take some time to work on silencing your negative thoughts.

Put your book by your bed tonight. In the morning before you get up, give yourself a few extra minutes to answer the following questions:

How did you feel when you woke up?

Did you get enough sleep? If no, why not?

If you dreamed, how did your dreams make you feel about yourself?

If a dream affected you negatively, what do you need to work on today to help you think more positively about yourself?

Answer these questions before you leave home:
How do you feel as you leave for school or work?

Do you feel motivated and clear about what you want to accomplish today? If not, what can you do to change this?

Answer these questions when you return home:

How did you feel during your day?

Did you plan all your activities for the day?   Yes   or   No

Were you able to stay with these plans?   Yes   or   No

If no, what happened?

What could you do next time to prevent this from happening?

> **Remember, repetition of behaviors and thoughts has an ongoing impact on your life. Whatever thoughts or actions you repeat over and over will become the thoughts or actions you have habitually.**

THE HEALTH CARE FIELD

Although the views in *Your Personal Trainer* come from a physician and a personal trainer/motivational expert, we often recommend treatment by other types of health care professionals as well. A fairly high percentage of the U.S.A. population sees medical providers in alternative medical fields. The following is a description of each of these professionals.

CHIROPRACTORS

Doctors of chiropractic medicine specialize in treatment of ailments that originate in the spine and nervous system. Chiropractors have had years of training somewhat similar to the training of physicians. They are particularly adept at treating musculoskeletal pain and ailments. Many also serve as primary care providers, although their treatments are confined to nonprescription treatment of disease.

If you have suffered an injury, it is important to seek treatment early-on. This helps to ensure proper healing, keep scar tissue formation to a minimum and reduce the chance of re-injury. As a general rule, if you do sustain an injury and your symptoms have not progressively improved within three days, it is important to seek teatment. Chiropractic, because, of its non-invasive approach, is one of the first avenues of therapy that could be sought out.

HOMEOPATHIC PHYSICIANS

These physicians are usually originally trained in standard medical schools and then go on to homeopathic medical training. Homeopathy uses nonprescription natural preparations that treat the whole patient as opposed to treating the disease itself. Much of the treatment involves giving tiny doses of substances to stimulate the body's immune responses.

HERBALISTS

These providers treat patients primarily through the use of herbal preparations and vitamins. All of these substances are found naturally occurring in the environment. One must be careful when using herbal products, because although they occur naturally, they are often given in doses that make them medicines. They can have all the risks and side effects of regular prescription medicines. Because they occur naturally they don't have to meet the same strict FDA requirements that prescription medications must meet. Herbalists can have many different levels of training. Check their credentials carefully before using their services.

ACUPUNCTURISTS

Acupuncture has become widely used to treat pain, injuries and other ailments. Acupuncturists can be physicians who went on to get additional training in acupuncture or they can be providers trained separately to provide acupuncture only. Training requirements vary depending on the state.

MASSAGE THERAPISTS

These specialists treat muscle spasms, trigger points, stress and injury. Hands on therapy of this nature can be very healing.

The following health professionals work closely with physicians and as such, are considered to be allied health care providers.

NURSE PRACTITIONERS

These providers are a well recognized part of the adjunct to medical profession. They typically are registered nurses who have gone on with at least two additional years of training in seeing patients and treating diseases. Many nurse practitioners have prescribing privileges for medications. They generally work under the supervision of a physician. Their approach focuses on wellness, prevention and patient teaching.

PHYSICIAN ASSISTANTS

Similar to nurse practitioners but often not certified to prescribe medications. They generally have two years of training after two to four years of prerequisites. Again they see patients under the supervision of a physician.

PHYSICAL THERAPISTS

Usually provide care as an independent entity but prescriptions must be written by a physician. They can be extremely helpful in treating injury and developing specific rehabilitation following an injury. They typically have a four year degree in physical therapy.

There are many professionals that can help you maintain a fit and well life.

DAY 21   **TODAY'S DATE**
TIME GOALS

*Were you able to achieve the three goals you set in Chapter Three?
If so, how?*

Goal 1:

Goal 2:

Goal 3:

For the rest of this book, continue to add one goal for each chapter. Use the skills you have applied so far to continue reaching your earlier goals and to reach your new ones, also. If you have struggled to achieve the goals you have set so far, ask yourself these questions:

Were your goals realistic?   *Yes*   *No*
Explain:

Did I procrastinate?   *Yes*   *No*
Explain:

Could I have used time better?   *Yes*   *No*
Explain:

As we've mentioned, it's difficult to change. You may have habits or
attitudes that prevent you from achieving your goals. Unless you
become aware of how this is happening, you will be frustrated in your
desire to make your life different. There are many ways to avoid
making changes. What are you doing to avoid making changes?
Check the behaviors that apply to you, then take a moment to think
of a way you can change these behaviors:

I sometimes watch too much television.
I could exercise instead of watching television.

How would this change help you achieve your goals?

I sometimes eat too much or use eating as a distraction.
I can do the following to reduce this:

How would this change help you achieve your goals?

I sometimes let others use my time when I need it for myself.
I can do the following to reduce this:

How would this change help you achieve your goals?

I sometimes perform less important tasks so I won't have to deal
with the more important ones. I can do the following to reduce
this:

How would this change help you achieve your goals?

CHAPTER FOUR

EXAMINE YOUR ENERGY LEVEL

BECOME AWARE OF HOW YOU ARE AFFECTED BY YOUR ENVIRONMENT

LEARN TO CONTROL THESE INFLUENCES

DAY 22   TODAY'S DATE:
EXAMINE YOUR ENERGY LEVEL

At the conclusion of Chapter Three, you examined some of the ways you may be keeping yourself from accomplishing your goals. It's important to stay aware of these. But it's also important to learn how to use your daily interactions and your environment to move yourself forward. In this chapter you'll begin to examine your daily energy levels, as well as your prevailing attitudes. It's these attitudes that can enhance your life or provide obstructions. Read and answer questions 1-50, on the next 5 pages and check the answers that apply to you now.

1.   *I have lots of energy and I look forward to each day.*
   ☐ Never   ☐ Seldom   ☐ Sometimes   ☐ Often   ☐ Always

2.   *I find a challenge exciting.*
   ☐ Never   ☐ Seldom   ☐ Sometimes   ☐ Often   ☐ Always

3.   *I show good judgment when I experience a difficult situation.*
   ☐ Never   ☐ Seldom   ☐ Sometimes   ☐ Often   ☐ Always

4.   *When I feel rushed and have deadlines to meet, I think of them as challenges.*
   ☐ Never   ☐ Seldom   ☐ Sometimes   ☐ Often   ☐ Always

5. *I believe that if I persist, I will overcome adversity.*
    ☐ Never   ☐ Seldom   ☐ Sometimes   ☐ Often   ☐ Always

6. *To avoid feeling overwhelmed, I set mental and physical goals that are attainable.*
    ☐ Never   ☐ Seldom   ☐ Sometimes   ☐ Often   ☐ Always

7. *I believe in my ability to remain faithful to my values.*
    ☐ Never   ☐ Seldom   ☐ Sometimes   ☐ Often   ☐ Always

8. *I feel motivated and determined.*
    ☐ Never   ☐ Seldom   ☐ Sometimes   ☐ Often   ☐ Always

9. *I can maintain my concentration to achieve a goal.*
    ☐ Never   ☐ Seldom   ☐ Sometimes   ☐ Often   ☐ Always

10. *To accomplish my goals, I keep myself ready and alert.*
    ☐ Never   ☐ Seldom   ☐ Sometimes   ☐ Often   ☐ Always

11. *I am happy with the decisions I make.*
    ☐ Never   ☐ Seldom   ☐ Sometimes   ☐ Often   ☐ Always

12. *When I feel stressed or depressed, I use exercise to relieve my feelings.*
    ☐ Never   ☐ Seldom   ☐ Sometimes   ☐ Often   ☐ Always

13. *When I feel overwhelmed or fatigued, I use a brief period of relaxation to rejuvenate myself.*
    ☐ Never   ☐ Seldom   ☐ Sometimes   ☐ Often   ☐ Always

14. *I eat a balanced intake of food.*
    ☐ Never   ☐ Seldom   ☐ Sometimes   ☐ Often   ☐ Always

15. *I take regular vacations.*
☐ Never   ☐ Seldom   ☐ Sometimes   ☐ Often   ☐ Always

16. *I enjoy interacting with others.*
☐ Never   ☐ Seldom   ☐ Sometimes   ☐ Often   ☐ Always

17. *I am able to achieve goals I have set for myself.*
☐ Never   ☐ Seldom   ☐ Sometimes   ☐ Often   ☐ Always

18. *I have the support I need.*
☐ Never   ☐ Seldom   ☐ Sometimes   ☐ Often   ☐ Always

19. *I use incentives to keep me focused on my goals.*
☐ Never   ☐ Seldom   ☐ Sometimes   ☐ Often   ☐ Always

20. *When I want to make changes in my life, I ask for help.*
☐ Never   ☐ Seldom   ☐ Sometimes   ☐ Often   ☐ Always

21. *I am happy with the choices I have made so far in my life.*
☐ Never   ☐ Seldom   ☐ Sometimes   ☐ Often   ☐ Always

22. *I stay motivated so I can accomplish my goals.*
☐ Never   ☐ Seldom   ☐ Sometimes   ☐ Often   ☐ Always

23. *I have the incentive, the knowledge and the support to change any unhealthy behaviors.*
☐ Never   ☐ Seldom   ☐ Sometimes   ☐ Often   ☐ Always

24. *I act contrary to my common sense and wants.*
☐ Never   ☐ Seldom   ☐ Sometimes   ☐ Often   ☐ Always

25. *I feel tired for no apparent reason.*
☐ Never   ☐ Seldom   ☐ Sometimes   ☐ Often   ☐ Always

26. *I feel confused and helpless.*
☐ Never ☐ Seldom ☐ Sometimes ☐ Often ☐ Always

27. *Because I feel uneasy around others, I avoid socializing.*
☐ Never ☐ Seldom ☐ Sometimes ☐ Often ☐ Always

28. *I have fears which prevent me from acting decisively.*
☐ Never ☐ Seldom ☐ Sometimes ☐ Often ☐Always

29. *Other people can make me feel rushed, stressed or worried.*

☐ Never ☐ Seldom ☐ Sometimes ☐ Often ☐Always

30. *There are times when I don't have the courage to act decisively.*
☐ Never ☐ Seldom ☐ Sometimes ☐ Often ☐ Always

31. *I feel restless and edgy.*
☐ Never ☐ Seldom ☐ Sometimes ☐ Often ☐ Always

33. *I have strong fears of situations I'm powerless to control or avoid.*
☐ Never ☐ Seldom ☐ Sometimes ☐ Often ☐ Always

35. *I feel I've reached a point where I need to make changes, but I'm not motivated.*
☐ Never ☐ Seldom ☐ Sometimes ☐ Often ☐ Always

36. *I have bowel problems - constipation, diarrhea, pain or bloating.*
☐Never ☐ Seldom ☐ Sometimes ☐ Often ☐Always

37. *I have brief periods of excessive agitation.*
☐ Never ☐ Seldom ☐ Sometimes ☐ Often ☐ Always

38.ㅤ*I have difficulty functioning as I have in the past.*
☐ Neverㅤㅤ☐ Seldomㅤㅤ☐ Sometimesㅤㅤ☐ Oftenㅤㅤ☐ Always

39.ㅤ*When I feel frustrated with my life, I don't want to face others. I would rather stay home to avoid any contact.*
☐ Neverㅤㅤ☐ Seldomㅤㅤ☐ Sometimesㅤㅤ☐ Oftenㅤㅤ☐ Always

40.ㅤ*I feel depressed.*
☐ Neverㅤㅤ☐ Seldomㅤㅤ☐ Sometimesㅤㅤ☐ Oftenㅤㅤ☐ Always

41.ㅤ*I find myself overeating when I feel stressed or depressed.*
☐ Neverㅤㅤ☐ Seldomㅤㅤ☐ Sometimesㅤㅤ☐ Oftenㅤㅤ☐ Always

42.ㅤ*I have a decreased sex drive.*
☐ Neverㅤㅤ☐ Seldomㅤㅤ☐ Sometimesㅤㅤ☐ Oftenㅤㅤ☐ Always

43.ㅤ*I find it hard to concentrate or feel motivated When I feel like this, I move too slowly to accomplish anything.*
☐ Neverㅤㅤ☐ Seldomㅤㅤ☐ Sometimesㅤㅤ☐ Oftenㅤㅤ☐ Always

44.ㅤ*I have trouble getting the same pleasure from my life I once got.*
☐ Neverㅤㅤ☐ Seldomㅤㅤ☐ Sometimesㅤㅤ☐ Oftenㅤㅤ☐ Always

45.ㅤ*I use alcohol or drugs as a means of relaxation.*
☐ Neverㅤㅤ☐ Seldomㅤㅤ☐ Sometimesㅤㅤ☐ Oftenㅤㅤ☐ Always

46.ㅤ*I have thoughts of harming myself or committing suicide.*
☐ Neverㅤㅤ☐ Seldomㅤㅤ☐ Sometimesㅤㅤ☐ Oftenㅤㅤ☐ Always

47.ㅤ*I feel inadequate.*
☐ Neverㅤㅤ☐ Seldomㅤㅤ☐ Sometimesㅤㅤ☐ Oftenㅤㅤ☐ Always

48.   I wish I had taken a different direction earlier in life.
☐ Never   ☐ Seldom   ☐ Sometimes   ☐ Often   ☐ Always

*49.   I don't have enough time for myself, my family or my
        friends.*
☐ Never   ☐ Seldom   ☐ Sometimes   ☐ Often   ☐ Always

50.   I have verbal disagreements with others.
☐ Never   ☐ Seldom   ☐ Sometimes   ☐ Often   ☐ Always

***Scoring these 50 questions will help you understand how
your emotions affect your approach to life. To score them,
write the correct points to the left of each number.***

Never .... 0 points   Often .... 3 points

Seldom .... 1 point..   Always .... 4 points

Sometimes .... 2 points

Add up your points for questions 1 – 23 and place the total here =
Add up your points for questions 24 – 50 and place the total here =

Add up the points for the first set of answers in Chapter One and
place the totals here.

Points for questions 1 – 23   +_____

Points for questions 24 – 50   - _____

Using the following graph, plot your four scores. You will be comparing your +(positive) scores and your -(negative) scores. Under your first score, place your (+) previous score from the start of the program above the line and your previous (-) score below the line. Use a dot (•)for the (+) score and an (x) for the (-) score. For today's score, do the same. Now connect the dots with one line and connect the x's with another.

Your First Score   Today's Score

			Extremely
80		80	
70		70	Highly
60		60	
50		50	
40		40	Moderately
30		30	
20		20	
10		10	Barely
0		0	
-10		-10	Ideally
-20		-20	
-30		-30	
-40		-40	Mildly
-50		-50	
-60		-60	
-70		-70	Overly
-80		-80	
			Excessively

Look at these lines. Have your scores changed since Chapter One? Have they gone down? Gone up? Stayed the same? These scores reflect two aspects of your energy levels.

POSITIVE LEVELS		NEGATIVE LEVELS	
Extremely	75+	Ideally	-1 – -24
Highly	55 – 74	Mildly	-25 – -35
Moderately	30 – 54	Overly	-36 – -50
Barely	0 – 29	Excessively	-51 – -80

*Compare your numbers to this chart and then
answer these questions:*
Before Chapter One, what was your positive energy level? _____
What is it now? _____
Before Chapter One, what was your negative energy level? _____
What is it now? _____

Your Personal Trainer has designed this graph so you can easily
see how influences in everyday life can affect your energy level.
You can use it as a baseline as you continue through this exercise
program.

What does each energy level mean?

+Level 4—Extremely Positive
If you are at this positive energy level, you are highly creative,
motivated, self-confident, sensitive and content with your life.

+Level 3—Highly Positive Energy
If you are at Level 3, you are usually fulfilled, content and moti-
vated. You do have occasional periods when you feel less content.
This is a state of greater than average positive energy.

+Level 2—Moderately Positive Energy
If you are at Level 2, you have intermittent periods of motivation,
happiness and creativity, but none of them are sustained. This is
a state of average positive energy, and a majority of people fall into
this category.

+Level 1—Barely Positive Energy

If you are at this energy level, you have little self-confidence and a lack of motivation, energy and self control. Level 1 is less than average positive energy.

-Level 1—Ideally Negative

If you are at Level 1, you are able to limit your negative feelings. These include feeling helpless, apprehensive and frustrated. You acknowledge these thoughts, but are able to notice them and move on. This is a state of above average negative energy.

-Level 2—Mildly Negative

This level is characterized by occasional periods of confusion, powerlessness, worry and uneasiness. However, for the most part, you are able to keep these feelings in check. This is the average amount of negative energy and many people function at this level.

-Level 3—Overly Negative

If you are at level 3 you have low stamina, are easily influenced by outside sources and are overly fearful. You feel powerless and frustrated, and have difficulty concentrating on what is important. This energy level can lead to depression, and the need to use food, drugs or alcohol to escape. This is a state of less than desirable negative energy and can prevent you from functioning productively and effectively in your daily life.

-Level 4—Excessively Negative

If you are at level 4, you are extremely frustrated, frightened and depressed. As a result, you find yourself restless, confused, uneasy and have strong feelings of helplessness. You have lost the desire to feel positive about your life and find yourself using food, alcohol or drugs to escape your feelings. You may find yourself feeling suicidal. If you think you are in this condition, seek medical attention.

WHAT IS YOUR GOAL?

Everyone has both positive and negative energy. Your goal is to move up one level for the positive and the same for the negative. For example, by answering all of the questions truthfully, you may have found you are moderately positive and mildly negative. This would put you in the majority of the population. Your goal will be to become highly positive and ideally negative.

You will find that many people you meet are moderately positive, but overly negative. The goal of this book is to try to help balance individuals' lives so they can become at least highly positive and mildly negative. If you are barely positive and overly negative, you may feel overwhelmed by trying to change your energy levels. However, always keep in mind that you are trying to just move one energy level at a time. When you achieve one goal, you can assess how you feel, and then challenge yourself to move to the next level. As with the rest of this program, the ways you choose to be as you change your attitudes and your habits should be thought of as life choices, not just temporary solutions.

Some of the hardest factors to overcome are outside influences that can affect your mood. To help you understand how you are affected, we have divided these factors into three components.

A. *Your knowledge or your beliefs . . .*
>   are firm convictions you consider to be true.
>   Information gained through experiences is knowledge.
B. *Feelings . . .*
>   are sensations involved in touching, emotional & intuitive.
>   are distinct mood or impression, a mental awareness.
>   can be about people or events you have experienced.
C. *Behavior . . .*
>   is how you act on your beliefs, information or feelings.

These three components will either help you to achieve your goals or they will get in your way. As you become aware of the ways in which you're influenced by your beliefs or feelings, you'll find yourself more able to take control of your life. Here are some examples of how these components can affect your life.

Example 1

If you feel that you're trapped in a body you don't like, you may find it difficult to make changes. Perhaps you've had negative experiences about this, such as derogatory comments from others. Your feelings and their remarks can drain you of the energy you need.

Example 2

To be able to accomplish a goal you've set for yourself, you must believe in your ability to achieve it. Outside influences that undermine this belief can make it difficult to stay on track. As you lose impetus, you become disconnected from your original intent. You also lose the ability to recognize signs of progress.

It's not always possible to control outside influences. Circumstances will affect you. But it is possible to recognize how you're being affected and in what ways you can protect yourself. We have integrated this self-awareness into your daily exercise routine. Using writing as a tool, you'll be able to see the negative and positive influences in your daily life. You'll see what lowers your energy level and what raises it. These observations and your commitment to health and exercise are the keys to improving your life.

Ways to increase your positive energy include:

- Working out
- Proper Nutrition
- Meditation
- Restful sleep
- Nurturing relationships

- Stretching
- Massage
- Positive thinking
- Written exercises
- Positive Visualization & Affirmation

Outside factors that can reduce your energy include:

- Violent television/movie images
- Abusive relationships
- Alcohol/drugs/overeating
- Friction with others
- Traffic
- Weather changes
- Concentration on guilt or regrets
- Noise

An increase in your energy level will be characterized by increased self-confidence and the ability to stay on the best course for yourself. A decrease in your energy level will manifest itself in a lack of focus and a feeling of self-doubt. The written exercises are keeping you aware of your daily energy changes and helping you control negative influences. You're learning to separate yourself from experiences such as bad days at work or heavy traffic, and not letting these lower your energy. As you continue, this process of identification and separation from negative influences will become easier.

For example, you may have answered "sometimes" to question #11, "happy with the decisions I make." With continued practice, you will be able to change your answer to "often." Question #29, "Other people may make me feel rushed, stressed or worried." You may be able to move from "often" to "sometimes."

> *As you go about your daily activities, concentrate on taking control of your life.*

AGE AS A HEALTH RISK FACTOR

Are you a man over 45 or a woman over 55? If so, your age gives you an additional risk factor for a heart attack. Rates of coronary artery disease are higher the older one gets. Women with early menopause not placed on estrogen are also at higher risk. Age is one more factor in taking seriously a long term exercise, weight reduction and healthy eating program.

WORKOUT: CARDIOMUSCULAR PREPARATION

Remember you want to keep in mind the following:

How you feel before starting your workout.

Why you're doing this workout.

How your responses compare to your previous ones.

If there is a difference. Why.

WALK/JOG   OR   BIKE

Time _____ *HR* _____   *Time* _____ *HR* _____
*Start*_____   *Start*_____
@ 6 min   _____   @   6 min   _____
@12 min   _____   @ 12 min   _____
@18 min   _____   @ 18 min   _____
@20 min   _____   @ 20 min   _____
*Stop*_____   *Stop* _____

Rest for sixty seconds before starting.

Lower Body Routine
1. Leg Curls and Leg Extension together / 1 set of 15 reps each (don't rest in between)
Smaller builds use 6 and 10 / 20 and 40 lbs
Larger builds use 15 and 20 / 40 and 50 lbs
Rest for 60 second and check your heart rate: _____

2. *Adductor individually / 1 set of 15 reps*
(don't rest between legs)
Smaller builds use 6 / 40 lbs
Larger builds use 16 / 60 lbs

3. *Stationary Lunges individually / 1 set of 15 reps*
   (don't rest between legs)
This exercise is performed without weights
Rest for 60 seconds and check your heart rate: _____

4. *One Leg Calf Raises - individually /1 set of 15 reps*
   (don't rest between legs)
This exercise is performed without weights
Rest for 30 seconds

Follow directions for the Mid Section Routine
(Chapter 9, pages 26 - 29))

Finish with a 20 second count stretch for all body parts.

Now that you are finished, reflect on these questions:

How did you feel during your workout?

Were you able to keep yourself motivated?

How do you feel now that your workout is finished?

Do you think and feel you're on your way to becoming
more fit?

Trainer's Comments and Suggestions:

DAY 23   TODAY'S DATE:
WORKOUT: CARDIOMUSCULAR PREPARATION

ROW		OR	WALK/ JOG	
Time ___ *HR* ___			*Time* ___ *HR* ___	
*Start*___			*Start*___	
@ 6 min	___		@ 6 min	___
@12 min	___		@ 12 min	___
@18 min	___		@ 18 min	___
@20 min	___		@ 24 min	___
*Stop*___			*Stop* ___	

Upper Body Routine

1. Bent Over Row and Push-ups or Lat Pull Downs and Chest Press Machine / 1 set of 15 reps for each (don't rest between)
Smaller builds use 12 and no lbs or 60 and 40 lbs
Larger builds use 30 and no lbs or 60 and 100 lbs
Rest for 30 seconds and check your heart rate: ___

2. Seated Lat Rows and Flat Bench Flies / 1 set of 15 reps for each
Smaller builds use 60 and 10 lbs
Larger builds use 80 and 25 lbs
Rest for 30 seconds

2. Lateral Deltoid Raises individually / 1 set of 15 reps (don't rest between reps)
Smaller builds use 5 lbs—Larger builds use 20 lbs

3. Triceps Kickbacks & Concentrated Biceps Curls/ 1 set of 15 reps (don't rest between)
Larger builds use 20 and 25 lbs—Smaller builds use 6 and 10 lbs
Rest for 30 seconds

4. Forearm Curls / 1 set of 15 reps
Smaller builds use 10 - 20 lbs —Larger builds use 20 - 40 lbs

Follow directions for the Mid Section Routine
(Chapter 9, Pages 26-29)

Finish with a 20 second count stretch for all body parts.

Make sure you are drinking enough water.

Trainer's Comments & Suggestions:

DAY 24   TODAY'S DATE:
MEDITATION: A TIME FOR SILENCE

Today is a day off from physical exercise. Instead, you will take the time to relax. As you go through the day, remember to notice how your energy is being affected by events and people. As you meditate, don't expect to feel any particular way. Your goal is to notice how being relaxed can affect and eventually control your low energy feelings. During your time of silence, free your mind of any concerns or anxieties. Maintain your time at 20 minutes. Choose meditation I or II.

GLYCOGEN REPLACEMENT

Following exercise, how quickly are glycogen stores replaced? Glycogen is the most readily available source of energy from the liver and muscle. Glycogen is fully restored within 24 hours after exercise if enough calories are consumed. Restoration of glycogen stores is greatest just after exercise. Therefore, you should start replacing glycogen stores immediately after heavy exercise by eating 1.5 to 2 gram/kg. of carbohydrate per kg of body weight. Another 1.2 to 2 grams/kg should be eaten an hour later. However, remember muscles, tendons and ligaments take two days to repair themselves from the minor traumas of routine exercise.

DAY 25 TODAY'S DATE:
WORKOUT: CARDIOMUSCULAR PREPARATION
Lower Body Routine

How do you feel before starting your workout?
Check all that apply to you.

☐ Motivated   ☐ Discouraged

☐ Excited   ☐ Dreading

☐ Pressed for time   ☐ Resigned

☐ Confident   ☐ Anxious

☐ Not sure   ☐ Ready and willing

☐ Clearheaded   ☐ Don't want to think about it

Do you know why you're doing this.   Yes   No   Explain:

WALK/JOG	**OR**	**BIKE**
Time _____ *HR* _____		*Time* _____ *HR* _____
*Start*_____		*Start*_____
@ 6 min _____		@ 6 min _____
@12 min _____		@ 12 min _____
@18 min _____		@ 18 min _____
@20 min _____		@ 20 min _____
*Stop*_____		*Stop* _____

Rest for 60 seconds before starting the next part of this workout.

Follow the lower body routine for Day 22. (pages 13-14)

Now that you have finished this workout, answer these questions:
How did you feel during your workout?

☐ Needed more energy   ☐ Energetic

☐ Distracted by negative thoughts   ☐ Powerful

☐ Could have gone on forever   ☐ Active

☐ My body and mind are adjusting   ☐ Happy

☐ I like how I'm feeling   ☐ Invigorated

Were you able to keep yourself motivated?   If so, how?
If not, why not?

How do you feel now that your workout is finished?

☐ Glad it's over   ☐ Rejuvenated

☐ Feel good about what I accomplished   ☐ Happy

☐ Can't wait until next time   ☐ Gratified

☐ Dreading next time   ☐ Renewed

☐ I wish I had started this long ago   ☐ Successful

☐ Now I understand why this is important ☐ Sore

Do you think and feel you're on your way to becoming more fit.
Yes   No   Explain:

Trainer's Comments and Suggestions:

Keep this book by your bedside and leave some extra time to
answer the following questions before you get out of bed.

BECOME AWARE OF HOW YOU ARE AFFECTED BY YOUR ENVIRONMENT

Answer these questions before you get out of bed in the morning:
How did you feel when you woke up?

Did you get enough sleep?   Yes   No   If no, why not?

How did your dreams make you feel about yourself?

If a dream or event affected you negatively, what do you need to work on today to help you think more positively about yourself?

It can be difficult to stay aware of how you think and feel during the day. The written exercises you have been doing should give you insight into the impact your daily influences have on your mood and attitude.

Another way to examine these influences is to think back over your day before you go to sleep. As you do this, you will find your sleeping hours can be used to change your perspective and even give you more control over your reactions to influences. You can't always control what happens to you in your life, but you can learn to control your reactions and the effect your reactions have on you.

EXAMINING THE INFLUENCES IN YOUR DAILY LIFE
Before you go to sleep tonight, think back over your day.
Can you recall moments that changed your thinking or feeling?
Did these events cause your energy to increase or lessen?

List the following:
Past experiences which are affecting you negatively now:

Past experiences which are affecting you positively now:

Present influences which are affecting you negatively now:

Present influences which are affecting you positively now:

Current goals which are most important and affecting you
positively now:

Current goals which are most important and affecting you
negatively now:

List the actions you took today to rid yourself of the results of the
negative influences:

List the actions you took today to reinforce the positive results of
past and present influences:

Past Influences:

Present Influences:

List one or more of these influences you experienced today that made you feel enthusiastic and excited:

Answer these questions before you leave home:
How do you feel as you leave for school or work?

Do you feel motivated and clear about what you want to accomplish today?

If not, what can you do to change this?

Answer these questions when you return home:
How did you feel during your day?

Did you plan all your activities for the day?   Yes   or   No
Were you able to stay with these plans?   Yes   or   No
If no, what happened?

What could you do next time to prevent this from happening?

Answer these questions at the end of your day:
How do you feel as the day is ending?

Did you accomplish what you wanted to accomplish?
Explain.

If you did, how can you reward yourself?

*If you weren't able to reach your goals, what steps could you take
to help yourself come closer tomorrow?*

This program encourages you to repeat positive behaviors over and
over. Just as negative behaviors can be maintained, so can positive
ones. As you learn to examine your daily life, including your
expectations and your accomplishments, you will see how you can
change unwanted patterns.

You can also learn to recognize the effect negative experiences are
having on you and therefore avoid feeling badly about yourself.
Always keep in mind that this process is ongoing.

When you've finished this exercise, have a good night's sleep.
In the morning there will be another written exercise to start your
day. The following exercise will help you become more aware of
how you are approaching your day. Place this book by your
bedside tonight.

DAY 26   TODAY'S DATE:
WORKOUT: CARDIOMUSCULAR PREPARATION
Upper Body Routine

Answer these questions before you get out of bed:
How did you feel when you woke up?

Did you get enough sleep?   Yes   No   If no, why not?

How did your dreams make you feel about yourself?

If a dream or event affected you negatively, what do you need to work on today to help you think more positively about yourself?

ROW		OR	WALK/JOG	
Time ____ *HR* ____			*Time* ____ *HR* ____	
*Start*____			*Start*____	
@ 6 min	____		@ 6 min	____
@12 min	____		@ 12 min	____
@18 min	____		@ 18 min	____
@20 min	____		@ 20 min	____
*Stop*_____			*Stop* _____	

Rest for 60 seconds

Follow the upper body routine for Day 23. (pages, 15-16)

Trainer's Comments and Suggestions:

DAY 27   TODAY'S DATE:
A DAY OFF
Today is a day off from physical exercise. Instead, you'll be learning more about how nutrition can affect your health and fitness.

READING FOOD LABELS
The food labeling that came out in May, 1994 can help you make better choices about what foods to eat. Reading labels is a crucial part of learning to eat well. Pay close attention to the saturated fat levels.

You can learn to calculate in your head approximately how many calories a food has, the grams of fat you are eating and the amount of fiber. Below is a sample of how to read and interpret a food label.

NUTRITIONAL FACTS

Serving Size	Will tell you individual serving of the food
Serving Container	Overall content of the food
Amount Per Serving	
Calories	The amount you will consume
Calories from fat	How many
Total fat	Listed in grams (g)
Saturated fat	
Polyunsaturated fat	
Mono-unsaturated fat	
Cholesterol	Listed in milligrams (mg.)
Sodium	Listed in milligrams (mg.)
Potassium	Listed in milligrams (mg.)
Total Carbohydrate	Listed in milligrams (mg.)
Dietary fiber	
Soluble fiber	
Sugars	
Other Carbohydrate	
Protein	

On some labels you may see a list of vitamins and the percentage listed within this food. You may also see the percentage of vitamins that is recommended for your daily intake.

You may also see that the Percent Daily Values are based on a 2,000 calorie food intake. Remember that your daily values may be higher or lower depending on your calorie needs.

What is the ideal % of calories from various types of foods? We recommend that the ideal food intake for an active exerciser consists of the following:

For each 1000 calories one should eat approximately:

150 grams carbohydrate

37 grams protein

28 grams of fat

$(150 \times 4 + 37 \times 4 + 28 \times 9 = 1000 \text{ cal})$

FUEL FOR ACTIVITY
The body produces energy by converting fat to fatty acids, protein to amino acids, and carbohydrates to sugar. Long duration (aerobic) exercise uses mostly fatty acids for energy, in addition to glycogen (complex carbohydrate) released from the liver and muscle.

As you train over a period of weeks, you will get better at using free fatty acids (fat) as fuel. Thus, you gradually become leaner with more exercise. Glycogen is the body's most immediate fuel source. It's used first for quick energy bursts, such as a sprint or weight lifting, by being released from liver and muscle tissue. Protein has little effect on performance, so protein is less necessary than carbohydrates and fat.

However, hemoglobin and red blood cell formation require iron plus protein. So, if you eat too little protein, hemoglobin cannot be made and anemia develops. Also, increased protein may be necessary when first starting out training, to allow for muscle and increase blood product formation.

MEDITATION:

Take the time to relax. As you go through the day, remember to notice how your energy is being affected by events and people. As you meditate, don't expect to feel any particular way. Your goal is to notice how being relaxed can affect and eventually control your low energy feelings. Choose meditation I or II (pages 1-30 or 1-31) and maintain your time at 20 minutes.

Keep this book by your bedside and allow for time
to do the following written exercises in the morning.

DAY 28 TODAY'S DATE:
LEARNING TO CONTROL INFLUENCES

This is not an easy task. Begin by noticing how you react to the many influences in your life.

Answer these questions before you get out of bed:
How did you feel when you woke up?

Did you get enough sleep? Yes No If no, why not?

How did your dreams make you feel about yourself?

If a dream or event affected you negatively, what do you need to work on today to help you think more positively about yourself?

It can be difficult to stay aware of how you think and feel during the day. The written exercises you have been doing will help give you insight into the impact your daily influences have on your mood and attitude.

Another way to examine these influences is to think back over your day before you go to sleep. As you do this, you'll find your sleep hours can be used to change your perspective and even give you more control over your reactions to influences. You can't always control what happens to you in your life, but you can learn to control your reactions and the effect your reactions have on you.

Examining the Influences in Your Daily Life

Before you go to sleep tonight, think back over your day.

Did you feel motivated and clear about what you wanted to accomplish today?

Can you recall moments that changed your thinking or feeling?

Positively

Negatively

Did these events cause your energy to increase or lessen?

What can you do to increase the positive and lessen the negative?

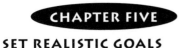

CHAPTER FIVE

SET REALISTIC GOALS

> ASSESSING YOUR BODY TYPE
> STAYING MOTIVATED
> GAINING PERSPECTIVE

DAY 29   TODAY'S DATE:
ASSESSING YOUR BODY TYPE
At the beginning of the book, we discussed the importance of knowing your body type. Understanding your body helps you set realistic and achievable goals for yourself. As you may remember, although there are three basic body types, most people are a combination of these types. In Chapter Five you will assess your body type. With this information, you will understand what can be changed and what can't.

There are three basic types:

ENDOMORPH
If you're an endomorph, you have a tendency to be stocky or round. Your bone structure is thick and you are either apple or pear shaped. Men tend more toward the apple shape, while women are more commonly pear shaped. An endomorph will have difficulty developing a trim and lean look. Your main obstacle to good health is fat retention. Set reasonable goals, based on what is possible, rather than an ideal you may never be able to attain.

ECTOMORPH
If you're an ectomorph, you have a thin light bone structure, long tenuous muscles and no problem with body fat retention. With consistent exercise you can develop a lean strong body, but it will be difficult for you to build large muscles.

MESOMORPH
If you're a mesomorph, you probably looked like an ectomorph as a teenager. As an adult, without exercising, you will either look similar to an ectomorph if you've remained slim over the years, or to an endomorph, if you're overweight. The distinction is that as you exercise, you can quickly build muscle. You can develop a defined and

muscular look. Fat retention can be a problem, but good eating habits will help you control this.

To summarize, an endomorph will always be an endomorph but can become more fit. An ectomorph will always look like an ectomorph but can firm up. A mesomorph, depending on whether or not he/she exercises, could look like an endomorph or an ectomorph. Again, recognize what body type you are and be realistic in working within those parameters. No matter what your body type, remember to:

- Stay motivated - remember why you want to make changes

- Keep an open mind and accept yourself

- Choose the right workouts for you

- Be consistent

- Stay with it, even when it's difficult to do so

WAIST-TO-HIP—RATIO
In Chapters One and Three you took measurements of yourself. In Chapter Five you will again measure your abdomen and your hips. Using these numbers, you'll determine their ratio as an indicator of whether or not your health is at risk. If you have a ratio of less than .80 for women and .90 for men you're in the normal group, with the lowest risk of heart problems. Ratios of .90 to .95 for men is border-line. Ratios above .8 for women and .95 for men increase your risk of heart disease. Men with ratios above 1.0 are at highest risk. To calcu-late your ratio, start by measuring your waist and your hips. You can either use a tape measure or a string and a yard stick. Waist is the smallest circumference below the ribs, but above the lateral pelvis measuring parallel to the floor. Hip is the largest circumference below the waist measuring parallel to the floor.
Record the numbers here: Abs_____ Hips_____

Now, divide the second number into the first. This is your ratio. Look back at your measurement at the start of the book and calculate your ratio. Have you shown improvements?

If you are feeling discouraged and haven't progressed as you'd hoped, answer the following questions:
In what ways haven't you followed your daily health goals?

Which behaviors are distracting you from staying motivated?

How have your attitudes and perceptions about yourself changed since you started this program?

Do you have physical or emotional barriers preventing you from achieving the changes you want to make? If so, what are they?

How will you overcome any negative beliefs you have about your body?

How has your attitude toward exercise changed since you started using this book?

Has the book helped to keep you motivated? If yes, in what ways?

SALT REQUIREMENTS

How much sodium does your body need? For a moderately active person, a minimum of 1100 mg. per day is required. The most intense exercise (i.e. Marathon running) requires as much as 10,000 mg. per day, but this is the exception.

The average American already ingests 3000 to 7000 mg. of salt per day, much of this hidden in snack foods, such as chips, and in meats, milk and seafood. So, unless you eat an unusually low level of salt, additional salt isn't needed for this exercise program. By the way, a hypertensive individual should restrict salt to under 2000 mg. per day.

WORKOUT: CARDIOMUSCULAR ENDURANCE
You will now move from cardiomuscular preparation workouts to cardiomuscular endurance workouts. The main difference between the two is an increase in the number of repetitions and the amount of weight in each exercise. Cardiomuscular endurance workouts will start preparing your body and mind for increased energy output.

WALK/JOG	OR	BIKE
Time _____ *HR* _____		*Time* _____*HR* _____
Start _____		*Start*_____
@ 6 min ____		@ 6 min ____
@12 min ____		@ 12 min ____
@18 min ____		@ 18 min ____
@20 min ____		@ 20 min ____
@24 min ____		@ 24 min ____
Stop _____		*Stop* _____

Go immediately to your first exercise

> *When two exercises are given together as one set,*
> *one set is comprised of the first and second exercise.*

LOWER AND UPPER BODY COMBINED ROUTINE

1. Leg Curls and Leg Extension
Smaller builds use 6 and 10 or 20 and 40 lbs
Larger builds use 15 and 20 or 60 and 80 lbs
2 sets of 12 reps for each exercise in this group
Rest for 60 seconds between sets and check your heart rate: ____

2. Adductor individually (don't rest between legs)
Smaller builds use 6 or 40   lbs
Larger builds use 16 or 60   lbs
2 sets of 12 reps
Rest for 30 seconds after the first set

3. Stationary Lunges individually (don't rest between legs)
This exercise is performed without weights - 2 sets for 12 reps
Rest for 60 seconds between sets and check your heart rate: _____

4. One Leg Calf Raises individually (don't rest between legs)
This exercise is performed without weights - 2 sets of 15 reps
Rest for 30 seconds after the first set

5. Bent Over Rows & Push-ups or Seated Lat Rows and Chest Press (don't rest between)
Smaller builds use 15 and no weights or 60 and 80 lbs
Larger builds use 30 and no weights or 80 and 100 lbs
2 sets of 12 reps each group
Rest for 60 seconds between sets and check your heart rate: _____

Are you drinking enough water?

6. Lat Pull Downs and Flat Bench Flies (don't rest between)
Smaller builds use 40 and   10 lbs
Larger builds use 80 and 20 lbs
2 sets of 12 reps each group
Rest for 60 seconds between sets and check your heart rate: _____

7. Lateral Deltoid Raises individually (don't rest between reps)
Smaller builds use 5 lbs
Larger builds use 20 lbs
2 sets of 10 reps
Rest for 60 seconds between sets and check your heart rate: _____

8. Triceps Kick Backs and Concentrated Biceps Curls (don't rest between)
Smaller builds use 6 and 10
Larger builds use 20 and 25 lbs
2 sets of 12 reps for each group
Rest for 60 seconds between sets and check your heart rate: _____

9. Forearm Curls / 2 sets of 12 reps
Smaller builds use 10 - 20 lbs
Larger builds use 20 - 40 lbs
Rest for 60 seconds between sets and check your heart rate: _____

10. Flat Back Leg Raises–2 sets of 25 reps

11. Flat Back Crunch Ups–2 sets of 25 reps

12. Side Crunches–2 sets of 25 reps on each oblique.

13. Flat Stomach Back Raises–2 sets of 25 reps

Finish with a 30 second count stretch for all body parts.

Trainer's Comments & Suggestions:

INJURIES
Job related injuries pose a major problem to workers, resulting in lost work days and high yearly income loss for individuals and companies.

Many of these injuries occur because people aren't in good enough physical shape to perform the job required of them. Muscles, tendons and ligaments become overused with a particular task and so break down, causing disability. A general conditioning and strengthening program, such as this one, may help to prevent injury. Many of the principles used in this book are the same as those used by rehabilitation therapists.

Staying with *Your Personal Trainer* on a long term basis should help you lessen injuries, both on the job and off.

> ***Take another look at how your actual routine compares to your goal times routine.***

DAILY ROUTINE

1. What time do you want to wake up?

    _____Goal time   _____Actual time

2. What time do you want to get out of bed?

    _____Goal time   _____Actual time

3. How long will it take you to eat your first meal?

    _____Goal time   _____Actual time

4. What time will you leave for work/school/other?

    _____Goal time   _____Actual time

5. What time will you arrive at work?

    _____Goal time   _____Actual time

6. What time will you start work?

    _____Goal time   _____Actual time

7. How long will it take you to eat your first snack?

    _____Goal time   _____Actual time

8. When will you work after you finish your snack?

    _____Goal time   _____Actual time

9. How long will your break be?

    _____Goal time   _____Actual time

10. How long will it take you to eat your lunch?

_____Goal time   _____Actual time

11. What time will you work after you finish your lunch?

_____Goal time   _____Actual time

12. How long will it take you to eat your second snack?

_____Goal time   _____Actual time

13. What time will you leave work?

_____Goal time   _____Actual time

14. How long will it take you to get home?

_____Goal time   _____Actual time

15. What time will you have dinner?

_____Goal time   _____Actual time

16. How much time will you spend watching television?

_____Goal time   _____Actual time

17. How much time will you take for meditation?

_____Goal time   _____Actual time

18. How much time will you devote to exercise?

_____Goal time   _____Actual time

19. How much time will you devote to family time?

_____Goal time   _____Actual time

20. How much time will you spend working at home?

_____Goal time   _____Actual time

21. How much time will you spend pleasure reading?

_____Goal time   _____Actual time

22. How much time will you spend in school study?

_____Goal time　　　_____Actual time

23. How much time will you devote to socializing with friends?

_____Goal time　　　_____Actual time

24. How much time will you spend doing chores?

_____Goal time　　　_____Actual time

25. What time will you go to bed?

_____Goal time　　　_____Actual time

Keep this book by your bed and give yourself
some extra time for tomorrow morning's written exercises.

DAY 30 　　　　TODAY'S DATE:
STAYING MOTIVATED

Today is a day off from physical exercise. However, before you get out of bed, do your written exercises. Working on these will help you stay motivated. These exercises are developed to help you stay aware of the various influences in your life and how they affect you. The way you act in any given situation is a result of influences that affect your daily life. These are: **Expectations, roles, physical environments, emotional environment, social environment** and **perceptions/attitude**. By reminding yourself of these every night, you will stay motivated so you can begin each day feeling more in control and conscious of your reactions as you go through your day.

Answer these questions before you get out of bed:
Did any of these influences help you toward a goal you have set?

Did any of these influences get in the way of a goal you have set?

Which ones got in the way of your goal?

What can you do to avoid this in the future?

Did you get enough sleep?   *Yes   or   No*
Did you dream about any of these goals?   Yes   or   No
If yes, how did they affect your feelings about yourself?

What do you need to work on today to help you think positively or maintain your positive feeling about yourself?

Answer these questions before you leave home:
Are you aware of any of the influences affecting you positively or negatively as you leave home? If yes, in what way?

Are you feeling motivated?   Yes   or   No
If no, how can you help yourself become motivated?

Answer these questions within an hour of leaving work or school:
How did you feel during your work or school day?

Did you plan all your activities for the day? Yes   or   No
Were you able to stay with your plans?   Yes   or   No
If no, what happened that got in your way?

Answer these questions at the end of your day:
How did you feel at the end of your school or work day?

Were you able to accomplish what you wanted to accomplish?
Yes   or   No   If no, why not?

If yes, how will you reward yourself?

If not, how can you make it possible to succeed tomorrow?

One of the challenges in trying to stay motivated and aware of how you think and feel, day after day, is the tendency to stay with the same thoughts. Each time there is a new experience, it's easier to have the same reaction you've always had. But to truly make changes, you must learn to recognize these patterns and try to replace them with thoughts that help you rather than hinder you.

One way to do this is to focus on what you're doing and why you're doing it. Then, stop the old behavior and replace it with the new. The repetition of new reactions will gradually result in new, more positive patterns. This is the basis for *Your Personal Trainer*: Recognizing what you want to change and allowing yourself the opportunity to change it.

In bed tonight, before you go to sleep, look back over your day and answer these questions:
What happened today that made you feel good about you?

What happened today as a result of one or more of the influences in your recent or distant past that affected you negatively?

What happened today as a result of one or more of the influences and is causing you to have either less or more energy at this moment?

What happened today that convinced you that you will not be able to overcome one or more of the influences?

What did you do today to help yourself because you were affected negatively by one or more of the influences?

Which of the influences gave you a positive attitude today?

Before you go to sleep tonight, have you balanced the positive and negative experiences? If you have, how have you done this?

As you look back over your answers, think about how your day could have been different. Could it have been more positive? Was it a good day? Did you learn something about yourself today?

Before you go to sleep, think about these five guidelines:

- Draw your own conclusions by evaluating and understanding what you see and hear.

- Be willing to act on your own evaluations and conclusions.

- Realize you can feel either positive or negative towards your life. The choice is yours.

- Learn to be adaptable. You may not always get what you want, when you want it.

- Learn the difference between thinking and knowing. Thinking is affected by your perceptions and knowing is a result of experience.

- Learn to use sound perception and judgment, then act on it.

EXERCISE INDUCED ASTHMA
Do you experience chest tightness, coughing or shortness of breath with exercise?

If you do, you may have exercise induced asthma. As much as 10% of the population has this, and over half of these people do not realize they have it. Exercise-induced asthma is characterized by restriction in the movement of air through the airways after 3 to 15 minutes of exercise. Occasionally, exercise-induced asthma occurs immediately after exercise or even several hours after exercise. Both men and women can have exercise-induced asthma.

DAY 31   TODAY'S DATE:
WORKOUT: CARDIOMUSCULAR ENDURANCE
Lower & Upper Body Combined Routine

WALK/JOG		OR	BIKE	
Time _____ *HR* _____			*Time* _____*HR* _____	
Start _____			*Start*_____	
@ 6 min	_____		@ 6 min	_____
@12 min	_____		@ 12 min	_____
@18 min	_____		@ 18 min	_____
@20 min	_____		@ 20 min	_____
@24 min	_____		@ 24 min	_____
Stop _____			*Stop* _____	

Go straight to your next exercise

Follow the lower & upper body combined routine for Day 29. (pages, 4-6)

Complete today's session by doing your stretching exercise.

Trainer's Comments & Suggestions:

MINERALS

The important minerals for exercise include zinc, copper, iron, chromium and selenium. Proper nutritional intake should provide enough of these for your exercise program. Minerals are typically found in meats, vegetables and milk products. In the high performance athlete, only iron and zinc can become deficient.

Iron is essential for the transport and use of oxygen. Most of the body's iron is present in the blood as hemoglobin or myoglobin. The recommended daily allowance is 10 mg. per day for adult men and post-menstruating women, and 15 mg. per day for menstruating women and teenagers.

Athletic training and exercise leads to an increased need for iron due to severe sweating and blood cell destruction by the pounding action of exercises such as running. Women can have major blood loss from menstruation. How can you tell if you have an iron deficiency or are anemic? If you are concerned about this, your doctor can measure your ferritin level and do a blood count. To get enough iron by food alone, eat plenty of meat, fish, poultry, dark leafy vegetables, dried fruits, whole grains and beans. Also, Vitamin C enhances the absorption of iron.

Women who are overly thin are often iron deficient. Being a vegetarian often adds to this deficiency. If you stop drinking milk, eating dairy products, and eating red meat your ferritin level will drop and you will be more likely to get injured. Men rarely become iron deficient. Runners with blood ferritin below 13 have twice the overuse injury rate of non runners. Being too thin also increases injury rate. Have your blood ferritin checked. If your level is less than 13, you need to improve your selection of foods or add iron supplements. Ideally ferritin should be over 24.

The recommended daily allowance of zinc is 15 mg. per day for men and 12 mg. per day for women. Lack of zinc can cause poor healing of wounds, poor growth and short stature, infertility and hair loss. Zinc is available in meat, liver, eggs and seafood. Whole grain products also contain small amounts of available zinc. Dietary fibers, although important in the prevention of diseases, may interfere with zinc absorption.

As a matter of interest, some people have found that the use of zinc lozenges can halve the amount of time they have cold symptoms and the severity of these symptoms.

Chromium is important in exercise, but is needed only in trace amounts. Our body gets plenty of chromium to meet our needs from the foods we eat. Chromium has received much attention from the media in recent years. However, the long term effects of a chromium supplement are not fully understood and chromium supplementation therefore is controversial.

Calcium - Though calcium does not play an immediate role in exercise, it is crucial in helping form strong bones and in keeping them strong. In fact, children ages 7 to 14 should take supplements of 1000 mg. of calcium tablets daily. Use of calcium will increase ultimate bone strength by age 21. Also, women of all ages benefit from taking 1500 mg. of calcium per day to prevent osteoporosis. Men may benefit also.

Tomorrow will be a day off from exercise.
Keep this book by your bed so you can answer
some questions before you get up in the morning.

DAY 32   TODAY'S DATE:
A DAY OFF

Today is another day off from physical activity. The questions below will help you focus on the goals you have set for yourself, and how you are feeling about them. If you need to, look again at the 6 influences that can affect how you feel and think daily.

Before you get out of bed, answer these questions:
How did you feel when you woke up?

I feel energetic, because:

I have no energy, because:

Did you get enough sleep?   Yes   or   No

How did your dreams affect you?

What do you need to work on today to make you feel good about yourself?

Answer these questions before you leave home:
How do you feel?

Are you feeling motivated?   Yes   or   No
If not, what can you do to help yourself feel motivated?

Answer these questions within an hour of leaving work or school:
How did you feel during your work or school day?

Was your day planned?   *Yes*   *or*   *No*
Were you able to stay with these plans?   *Yes*   *or*   *No*
If not, why not?

How did you feel at the end of your school or work day?

Were you able to reach your goals?   *Yes*   *or*   *No*
If so, how will you reward yourself?

If not, what changes can you make tomorrow so you will be able to reach them?

Remember, it's important to remain aware of how you feel and think during the day. This awareness makes it easier for you to feel in control of your life. Your awareness of how you feel and think, and why you do what you do will help you change old habits into new ones.

Answer these questions in bed tonight:
What experiences did you have today that caused you to change your
feeling or thinking to make you feel either more positive or more
negative?

Positive Experience:

Negative Experience:

IRREGULAR MENSES
Women who exercise hard may develop irregular menses, due to
disruption of the normal hormonal controls. This may be compounded
by getting down to lower weight with exercise and sometimes by
stress.

Menses may disappear completely (for more than 6 months) in some
women or may become quite irregular in timing and duration in others.
If you have had or develop such problems, you should see your doctor
to assure there are no other factors causing the problem. Irregularity or
absence of menses over many years can increase the risk of uterine
cancer. Treatment is available with estrogen and progesterone.

DAY 33   TODAY'S DATE:
WORKOUT: CARDIOMUSCULAR ENDURANCE

Lower and Upper Body Combined

Before beginning your workout, answer these questions:

How do you feel before starting your workout? (Check one or more)

☐ Motivated   ☐ Discouraged

☐ Excited   ☐ Dreading

☐ Pressed for time   ☐ Resigned

☐ Confident   ☐ Anxious

☐ Not sure   ☐ Ready and willing

☐ Clear-headed   ☐ Don't want to think about it

I know why I'm doing this (Check one)   Yes   No   Explain:

How do these answers compare to your previous ones?
If there is a difference, why?

WALK/JOG **OR**	**BIKE**
Time _____ *HR* _____	*Time* _____ *HR* _____
Start _____	*Start* _____
@ 6 min _____	@ 6 min _____
@12 min _____	@ 12 min _____
@18 min _____	@ 18 min _____
@20 min _____	@ 20 min _____
@24 min _____	@ 24 min _____
Stop _____	*Stop* _____

Go straight to your next exercise

Are you drinking enough water?

Go immediately to your first exercise.

Follow lower & upper body combined routine for Day 29, (pages, 4-6)

Complete today's session by doing your stretching exercise.

How did you feel during the exercises? (Check one or more answers)

☐ I needed more energy ☐ I had too many negative thoughts

☐ I could have gone on forever ☐ I felt good after it was over

☐ I just wasn't interested today ☐ I need a partner

☐ I felt energetic ☐ I felt powerful

☐ What an invigorating feeling ☐ It's good to have my body active

Were you motivated?   *Yes*   *No*   *If not, why not?*

If you were, what was motivating you?

How do you feel now that your workout is finished?

☐ Glad it's over ☐ Joyful

☐ Feel good about what I accomplished ☐ Poised

☐ Can't wait until next time ☐ Gratified

☐ I wish I'd started this long ago ☐ Rejuvenated

☐ Now I understand why this is important ☐ Successful

Did the exercise make you feel more positive? Why or why not?

Trainer's Comments & Suggestions:

MEDITATION: A TIME FOR SILENCE

Today you'll be combining physical exercise with your meditation routine. Your goal for this time is to try to free your mind of any distracting thoughts. Give yourself this opportunity to step away from your life and gain perspective on how you are feeling and what affects those feelings. Pay attention to what you let dominate your mind and what affects those experiences are having on your ability to think clearly. Increase your time to 25 minutes. Choose meditation I or II

EXERCISE & EFFICIENCY

Did you know that exercise increases your efficiency at other times of the day?

Exercise calms the mind, yet increases energy for accomplishing tasks. This may not be apparent at first, but after weeks of exercise you should find improvement in your work or study efficiency and your overall well-being. Employers should encourage their employees to start an exercise routine and see the positive effects on job efficiency and morale.

DAY 34   TODAY'S DATE:
GAINING PERSPECTIVE

Today is another day off from physical exercise. Instead, you will take the time to understand why it is important to gain perspective on what you do each day. Take this time to look at the ways your daily behaviors and decisions may be lowering your energy.

Look again at these influences: **Expectations, roles, physical environment, emotional environment, social environment** and **perceptions/attitude**. How do these affect you each day? As you become more able to recognize the interplay between these influences and how you are feeling and thinking, you will find it easier to manage negative feeling and thoughts.

Throughout today, watch for changes in your feelings and thoughts. When do you feel invigorated or excited? Why are you allowing negative self-talk to take over your consciousness? When do you feel slowed down or drained? Which of these influences are causing these reactions? Explain your reactions to these.

Expectations

Roles

Physical environment

Emotional environment

Social environment

Perceptions/Attitude

ASTHMA

Exercising in dry, cold air can trigger asthma as can air pollutants and allergens. Some people get only a cough or chest tightness. Diagnosis should be made by a doctor. As much as 10% of the population has exercise-induced asthma and over half of these people do not realize they have it.

Treatment is best done with inhalants before exercise and with trying to avoid exercise in cold dry air. Exercise in a warm, moist environment and avoid mouth breathing. Also, general conditioning gradually tends to improve the asthma. For an athletic event, one can warm up 45 minutes before the event. There is typically a window of time before exercising, lasting an hour during which one is less likely to develop symptoms.

DAY 35   TODAY'S DATE:
WORKOUT: CARDIOMUSCULAR ENDURANCE

Lower and Upper Body Combined Routine

WALK/JOG   OR   BIKE

Time _____ *HR* _____		*Time* _____ *HR* _____	
Start _____		*Start* _____	
@ 6 min	_____	@ 6 min	_____
@12 min	_____	@ 12 min	_____
@18 min	_____	@ 18 min	_____
@20 min	_____	@ 20 min	_____
@24 min	_____	@ 24 min	_____
Stop _____		*Stop* _____	

Go straight to your next exercise

Follow the lower & upper body combined routine for Day 29.
(pages, 4-6)

Complete today's session by doing your stretching exercise.

Trainer's Comments & Suggestions:

ARTHRITIS & EXERCISE

For people with arthritis, exercise is critical. Long periods of abstinence from physical activity exacerbates the musculoskeletal consequences of the disease.

If you have arthritis, you may have felt that rest would be the best treatment for it. But, as most physicians will tell you, people with arthritis will benefit from proper exercise without experiencing worsening symptoms. In fact, exercise may help in slowing the progress of the disease.

What types of exercises should you do if you have arthritis?
The choice of exercise will depend partly on the stage of the disease, the pattern of joint involvement and the availability of helpful instructions. Both aerobic and strengthening exercises have been shown to be beneficial.

Many of the exercises in this book are helpful for people with arthritis, but for those with significant effects, assistance must be sought from a qualified physician or physical therapist to best determine how to use this exercise program. In general, people with arthritis respond well to aerobic exercise, such as walking and aquatics. Isometric exercises produce moderate gains in strength and offer the greatest protection to arthritic joints.

If you have arthritis keep these points in mind:

- A full range of motion is necessary before beginning strengthening exercises.

- Exercise should begin slowly and be monitored carefully.

- High impact exercise, such as running and jumping, should be avoided unless arthritis is minimal.

- Regular exercise decreases daily pain symptoms, as well as joint swelling and stiffness.

The addition of an anti-inflammatory medication prior to exercise or on a regular basis also helps to decrease pain and inflammation from arthritis. Overall, if you have arthritis, a regular exercise routine improves endurance, decreases pain, helps self-confidence and decreases depression.

CHAPTER SIX

MAKE PERMANENT CHANGE

CONTINUE TO EVALUATE
CONTINUE TO EXERCISE
CONTINUE TO RECOGNIZE YOUR PATTERNS

DAY 36   TODAY'S DATE:
CONTINUING TO EVALUATE

In order to make permanent changes in your lifestyle routine, it's important for you to continue to evaluate your patterns. Do you procrastinate? Do you spend time with your family?

Chapter Six is a continuation of the physical exercises, writing exercises and meditation routine you've been following. As you follow the daily routines, keep these five principles in mind.

- Recognize that what you see and hear affects how you feel about yourself and others.

- Look closely at your strengths and weaknesses.
  Be realistic but kind.

- Identify the reasons for your high and low energy levels by noticing your physical environment, personal relationships and roles.

- Organize your schedule so you have time for meditation as well as physical exercise. You need both.

- Develop healthy eating habits.

   These five principles will help you stay aware of how your environment is affecting you.

WORKOUT: CARDIOMUSCULAR ENDURANCE
Lower Body Routine

W A L K / J O G	OR	B I K E

Time _____ *HR* _____	*Time* _____ *HR* _____
Start _____	*Start* _____
@ 6 min _____	@ 6 min _____
@12 min _____	@ 12 min _____
@18 min _____	@ 18 min _____
@20 min _____	@ 20 min _____
@24 min _____	@ 24 min _____
@30 min _____	@ 30 min _____
*Stop*_____	*Stop* _____

Are you drinking enough water?

Go immediately to your first exercise

1. Flat Back Leg Raises - 1 set - 50 reps

2. Flat Back Crunch Ups - 1 set - 50 reps

3. Side Crunches - 1 set - 50 reps for each oblique

4. Flat Stomach Back Raises - 1 set - 50 reps

5. Leg Curls and Leg Extension (don't rest between legs)
Smaller builds use 15 - 40 lbs
Larger builds use 25 - 60 lbs
1 set of 20 reps on each exercise
Rest for 60 seconds and check your heart rate: _____

6. Adductor individually (don't rest between legs)
Smaller builds use 10 - 40 lbs
Larger builds use 20 - 60 lbs
1 set of 20 reps

7. Alternating Leg Lunges (don't rest between legs)
This exercise is performed without weights   1 set of 20 reps
Rest for 60 seconds and check your heart rate: _____

8. One Leg Calf Raises individually (don't rest between legs)
This exercise is performed without weights
1 set of 20 reps

Finish with the stretching routine

Trainer's Comments & Suggestions:

TREADMILL STRESS TEST
What is a treadmill stress test? This test drives your heart rate up as
you exercise. During this time, your cardiogram is monitored, recording the electric current coming from your heart. By looking at the
changes in the electrical pattern with exercise, one can make predic-
tions about whether or not there is significant coronary artery disease.
The test is a very useful predictor in people with risk factors of coronary disease. Should everyone have a treadmill stress test? One would
think so, but the answer is no. Surprised? Why shouldn't everyone
have one? The treadmill stress test is not a perfect test.

As the number of risk factors go up (i.e. increasing age, family history,
hypertension, diabetes, etc.), the test becomes more accurate and
predictive because the chance that one has disease is greater. In someone with no risk factors, the chances of real heart disease is low, but
the chances of a wrong test is still present. So if you take a 35 year old
man with no risk factors and you get a treadmill test with an abnormal
result, there is more than an 80% chance that the test is wrong. This
can lead to more tests, possible risk and much worry. On the other
hand, a 50 year old male, hypertensive smoker whose father died at
age 51 of a heart attack should have a treadmill test.

WHO SHOULD TAKE A TREADMILL TEST?

In general, men over 40 years old and women over 50 years old should have a treadmill test prior to engaging in a strenuous exercise (i.e. jogging, racquetball, tennis, uphill biking, etc.). This recommendation includes both lower and higher risk individuals. Younger people who have high risk factors should have a treadmill test prior to strenuous exercise. Anyone, regardless of age, with symptoms of a heart or chest problem should have a treadmill test prior to engaging in even moderate exercise.

Healthy, low coronary risk people, of any age, without symptoms, can generally participate in moderate (i.e. walking, light biking) exercises without prior treadmill stress testing. Many of the exercises in this book fall into the strenuous category. The above are general guidelines from the American College of Sports Medicine, 1996. Consult your own physician to determine your individual needs.

DAY 37   TODAY'S DATE:
WORKOUT: CARDIOMUSCULAR ENDURANCE
Upper Body Routine

ROW / WALK / JOG	OR	BIKE

Time _____ *HR* _____   *Time* _____ *HR* _____
Start _____   *Start* _____
@ 6 min   _____   @ 6 min   _____
@12 min   _____   @ 12 min   _____
@18 min   _____   @ 18 min   _____
@20 min   _____   @ 20 min   _____
@24 min   _____   @ 24 min   _____
@30 min   _____   @ 30 min   _____
 Stop _____   *Stop* _____

Make sure you are drinking enough water.

Rest for 60 seconds, then start:

1. Flat Back Leg Raises - 1 set - 50 reps

2. Flat Back Crunch Ups - 1 set - 50 reps

3. Side Crunches - 1 set - 50 reps for each oblique

4. Flat Stomach Back Raises - 1 set - 50 reps

5. Lat Pull Downs and Chest Press (don't rest between)
Smaller builds use 30 - 60 and 10 - 20 lbs
Larger builds use 60 - 100 and 95 - 135 lbs
1 set of 20 reps on each exercise
Rest for 30 seconds and check your heart rate: _____

6. Seated Lat Rows and Flat Bench Flies (don't rest between)
Smaller builds use 40 - 60 and 10 - 20 lbs
Larger builds use 60 - 100 and 20 - 40 lbs
1 set of 20 reps on each exercise
Rest for 60 seconds and check your heart rate: _____

7. Lateral Deltoid Raises individually (don't rest between)
Smaller builds use 5 - 12 lbs
Larger builds use 15 - 20 lbs
1 set of 20 reps

8. Triceps Push Down and Concentrated Biceps Curls
(don't rest between)
Smaller builds use 20 - 40 and 10 - 20 lbs
Larger builds use 40 - 60 and 20 - 30 lbs
1 set of 20 reps for each exercise

It's important to finish your workout with stretching routine.

Trainer's Comments & Suggestions:

INFLAMMATION

Preventing inflammation after exercise can be important in avoiding injury and decreasing pain. Ice is nature's anti-inflammatory. An area of swelling should be iced for 15 to 20 minutes. You can use a bag of frozen peas or corn over an overused area you suspect might develop trouble. Ice may also be massaged in, using a bare ice cube. With few exceptions, ice is better than heat.

Nonsteroidal, anti-inflammatory medication, both prescription and over the counter, provide an effective way of decreasing inflammation. Different medications have varying effects on different individuals. These medications relieve pain, as well as decreasing inflammation.

DAY 38   TODAY'S DATE:
MEDITATION ROUTINE: A TIME FOR SILENCE

Today is a day off from physical exercise. Instead, keep eating a balanced intake of food and take time for meditation. As you go through the day, remember to notice how your energy is being affected by events and people. As you meditate, don't expect to feel any particular way. Your goal is to notice how being relaxed can eventually give you more energy. During your time of silence, free your mind of any concerns or anxieties. Maintain your time at 25 minutes. Choose meditation I or II.

CARBO LOADING

Carbohydrate loading means taking in high amounts of carbohydrates and decreasing exercise for several days before an event. This increase results in an elevation of the muscle glycogen stores.

If you carbo load for three days, the muscle carbohydrate stores double. Higher muscle glycogen increases performance and decreases muscle recovery time in exercise such as long distance running.

For the purposes of *Your Personal Trainer*, you won't need to do any carbo loading. Maintain a balanced intake of food as has been previously discussed. However, if you're doing our program in combination with training for an event (i.e. a 10k race), you may improve your performance by carbo loading as described here.

DAY 39   TODAY'S DATE:
WORKOUT: CARDIOMUSCULAR ENDURANCE
Lower Body

WALK/JOG   OR   BIKE

Time _____ *HR* _____		*Time* _____ *HR* _____	
Start _____		*Start* _____	
@ 6 min	_____	@ 6 min	_____
@12 min	_____	@ 12 min	_____
@18 min	_____	@ 18 min	_____
@20 min	_____	@ 20 min	_____
@24 min	_____	@ 24 min	_____
@30 min	_____	@ 30 min	_____
Stop _____		*Stop* _____	

Are you drinking enough water?

Follow lower body routine for Day 36. (page, 2-3)
It's important to finish with the stretching routine.

Trainer's Comments & Suggestions:

Are you paying attention to your daily routine?

DAILY ROUTINE

1. What time do you want to wake up?

_____Goal time   _____Actual time

2. What time do you want to get out of bed?

_____Goal time   _____Actual time

3. How long will it take you to eat your first meal?

_____Goal time   _____Actual time

4. What time will you leave for work/school/other?

_____Goal time   _____Actual time

5. What time will you arrive at work?

_____Goal time   _____Actual time

6. What time will you start work?

_____Goal time   _____Actual time

7. How long will it take you to eat your first snack?

_____Goal time   _____Actual time

8. After you finish your snack, when will you work?

_____Goal time   _____Actual time

9. How long will your break be?

_____Goal time   _____Actual time

10. How long will it take you to eat your lunch?

_____Goal time   _____Actual time

11. What time will you work after you finish your lunch?

_____Goal time   _____Actual time

12. How long will it take you to eat your second snack?

_____Goal time   _____Actual time

13. What time will you leave work?

_____Goal time   _____Actual time

14. How long will it take you to get home?

_____Goal time   _____Actual time

15. What time will you have dinner?

_____Goal time   _____Actual time

16. How much time will you spend watching television?

_____Goal time   _____Actual time

17. How much time will you take for personal quiet time?

_____Goal time   _____Actual time

18. How much time will you spend exercising?

_____Goal time   _____Actual time

19. How much time will you devote to family time?

_____Goal time   _____Actual time

20. How much time will you devote to work/study?

_____Goal time   _____Actual time

21. How much time will you spend in pleasure reading?

_____Goal time   _____Actual time

22. How much time will you devote to school/study?

_____Goal time   _____Actual time

23. How much time will you spend socializing with friends?

_____Goal time   _____Actual time

24. How much time will you devote to chores?

_____Goal time   _____Actual time

25. What time will you go to bed?

_____Goal time   _____Actual time

DAY 40 TODAY'S DATE:
WORKOUT: CARDIOMUSCULAR ENDURANCE
Upper Body Routine

R O W / W A L K / J O G OR B I K E

Time _____ *HR* _____		*Time* _____ *HR* _____	
Start _____		*Start* _____	
@ 6 min	_____	@ 6 min	_____
@12 min	_____	@ 12 min	_____
@18 min	_____	@ 18 min	_____
@20 min	_____	@ 20 min	_____
@24 min	_____	@ 24 min	_____
@30 min	_____	@ 30 min	_____
Stop _____		*Stop* _____	

Are you drinking enough water?

Rest for 60 seconds before starting the next exercises.

Follow the upper body routine for Day 37 (pages, 4-5)
It's important to finish with the stretching routine.

Trainer's Comments & Suggestions:

DAY 41   TODAY'S DATE:
A DAY OFF
Today is a day off from physical workouts. Instead, you'll concentrate on increasing your knowledge about general health.

UNDERSTANDING CHOLESTEROL
Cholesterol can most easily be understood as the sum of three parts:

LDL (Low density lipoprotein) or "bad" cholesterol, HDL (high density lipoprotein) or "good" cholesterol and TGL (triglycerides), a form of fat in the bloodstream. Total cholesterol = LDL + HDL + TGL/5

In assessing your cholesterol risk, it's important to know each part rather than just the total count. If you haven't had your level checked in the past year, we suggest you do this, noting each number.

WHAT IS A GOOD TOTAL CHOLESTEROL NUMBER?
Ideally, your total cholesterol number should be less than 200. The lower it is, the better. 200-240 is borderline high cholesterol. Above 240 is high blood cholesterol.

But this doesn't give the whole picture. Your HDL is extremely important. The higher the HDL, the lower the risk of coronary artery disease and heart attacks. HDL should be approximately above 40 for men and above 45 for women. Less than 35 for either is considered definitely low. HDL above 60 actually becomes a "negative risk factor", and can negate one of the positive risk factors such as hypertension. Low HDL, especially below 35, becomes a significant positive factor in increasing one's risk of heart disease.

HOW CAN YOU RAISE YOUR HDL?
Your starting HDL is affected most by heredity. But there are ways you may be able to raise it beyond this number. Exercise will usually increase it by small amounts (3-5 points). Both weight reduction and small amounts of alcohol can increase HDL by 1 or 2 points. Smoking can decrease your HDL. Small increases are more important than they may appear - every point increase in HDL decreases your heart attack risk by 2%.

If you have low HDL, especially below 35, you should seek your doctor's advice. Prescription medicine and niacin can significantly raise HDL. But because of the possible side affects, these measures are usually reserved for men over 35 and postmenopausal women. Niacin must be taken in medicinal doses of 1.5-4 grams to be effective. At these doses it can occasionally irritate the liver, so blood tests must be carefully monitored. Don't take it without your doctor's help.

LDL Cholesterol or "Bad" Cholesterol
Simply stated, the higher your LDL, the greater your risk of heart disease.

Less than 130 — Normal
130-159 — Borderline high risk LDL cholesterol
160 or greater — High risk LDL cholesterol

The main contributors to high LDL are an unhealthy nutritional intake and heredity. Since you can't change heredity, the best ways to reduce LDL are to change your eating habits and lose weight if you need to do that. Exercising and adding fiber to your intake can also help reduce this number. Every one point decrease represents a 2% decrease in heart disease risk. Several prescription medicines are available and these may help reduce your LDL, which in turn will lower your total cholesterol.

The foods you consume play a significant role in LDL levels for some people. A significant change in your eating habits can dramatically lower LDL levels for these individuals. Yet for many others, LDL is mostly hereditary, and no matter how hard they work on it, LDL stays about the same. This fact can be quite frustrating, but fortunately modern medications work well if indicated.

Most people should aim to achieve an LDL of 130 or less. In the healthy individual, medication is indicated if a change in food consumption and weight loss have failed to bring the LDL below 190 (unless HDL is greater than 60).

If one has two or more additional risk factors for coronary disease (but no disease yet), medication is indicated if food consumption and weight loss have failed to bring the LDL below 160.

However, if one already has coronary artery disease, doctors must be more aggressive and get LDL below 100 to prevent building additional artery plaque.

Triglycerides (TGL)
Triglycerides can best be thought of as fat circulating in the bloodstream. This fat can play an important role in causing coronary heart disease. In some people, high TGL is hereditary and every family member has this problem. For these people, the TGL stays high no matter how healthy their eating habits. However, a bad intake makes their TGL even worse. For many people, though, high TGL is directly related to an intake high in fat. For these people, improving proper nutrition can lower their TGL within days. In contrast, it can take months to improve your HDL or LDL with proper intake or exercise.

Below 80 — Ideal TGL
Below 140 — Satisfactory TGL
Above 140 — Elevated TGL, needs improvement

Extremely high TGL (above 500) can injure the pancreas over time, causing a life threatening disease called pancreatitis. Therefore, this kind of TGL reading requires more urgent attention. The best way to begin lowering your TGL is by eating less fat, particularly saturated fat. If this doesn't work, again niacin and prescription medicine can be helpful.

*The goal for your cholesterol level should be
to make it the healthiest you can:*

Raise HDL with exercise and, if necessary, with niacin or prescription medication (ideal: HDL above 60; acceptable: HDL above 40)

Lower LDL with proper intake, fiber and, if necessary, medication (goal of less than 160, but ideal of less than 130)

Lower TGL with proper intake first and, if necessary, with medication (ideal of less than 140)

The numbers *Your Personal Trainer* has given you are averages. To find the exact values for you, based on your cholesterol level and your risk factors, consult your physician. Medication is effective in lowering cholesterol in every age group. However, in younger patients such as men under 35 and premenopausal women, doctors tend to reserve it for those with other risk factors, such as diabetes, FmHx (family history), smoking or HTN(hypertension), and for those with extremely severe elevations of LDL. If you've worked hard on your cholesterol and haven't been able to make a change, consult your doctor. Or, send your numbers on the back of a postcard to us at demor@pacbell.net and an analysis will be done for you.

Include the following information:
Sex_____   Age_____   HDL____   LDL____   TGL____
Total cholesterol_____
Smoker?_____ Diabetes?_____
Hypertension Hx_____
FmHx of heart attack_____   Who?_____   Age?_____
What have you tried so far?

Changes in your food intake?   Yes   No
If yes, what have you done?

Except for those people with purely hereditary high cholesterol, what you eat will affect your cholesterol level. To improve yours, follow these rules:

1.   Keep saturated fat to no more than 8-10% of total calories.

2. No more than 30% of total calories should come from fat

3. Keep cholesterol intake to less than 30 mg./day

4. Be patient – it can take 6 months to lower your cholesterol.

If your levels are still not what you want after 6 months, reduce your saturated fat to 7% of calories and your cholesterol to 20 mg./day.

DAY 42   TODAY'S DATE:
CONTINUE TO RECOGNIZE YOUR PATTERNS
It's difficult to stay aware all day of how you're feeling. Your life becomes busier and busier, and you must move quickly from one situation to another. There are problems to solve, other people to deal with, goals to accomplish. Taking the time to sort this information and feel its effects on you can be daunting or even impossible at times. But as you practice looking back over your day and looking ahead, you will begin to have moments of awareness that didn't exist previously. This is progress. It may be slow, it may stop and start, but if you persist, you will find your awareness increasing. As it increases, you will feel more in control of your life.

EXAMINE THE INFLUENCES IN YOUR DAILY LIFE
Before you go to sleep tonight, think back over your day. Can you recall moments that changed your feeling and thoughts? Did these events cause your energy to increase or lessen?

List the following:

Past experiences which are affecting you negatively now:

Past experiences which are affecting you positively now:

Present influences which are affecting you negatively now:

Present influences which are affecting you positively now:

Current goals which are most important to you and are affecting you positively now:

Current goals which are most important to you and are affecting you negatively now:

List the actions you took today to rid yourself of the results of the negative influences:

List the actions you took today to reinforce the positive results of past and present influences:

Past:

Present:

List one or more of these influences you experienced today that made you feel enthusiastic and excited, and tell why:

When you find yourself reacting to a situation in a way you don't like, you can choose to notice and learn.

When you've finished this exercise, have a good night's sleep.

EXERCISE FOR THE ELDERLY

Is it important? Definitely. As one ages, daily exercise continues to be important. *Your Personal Trainer* can be used effectively for older people, as well as for the young. Exercise keeps muscles and joints working at their most comfortable level. It can decrease the pain and stiffness caused by arthritis, and help prevent osteoporosis in women.

Other possible benefits of exercise include prevention of heart attacks by decreasing plaque formation in blood vessels, decreasing LDL cholesterol, increasing HDL cholesterol, preventing obesity and decreasing hypertension.

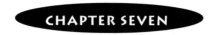

CHAPTER SEVEN

STAY ON TRACK

EXAMINE YOUR APPROACH TO EXERCISE
STAY AWARE

DAY 43 TODAY'S DATE:

EXAMINE YOUR APPROACH TO EXERCISE

There are four fitness types: Beginner, Ambivalent, Obsessive and Balanced. Which are you? Is this the same type you were when you started this program? Just to review:

BEGINNER

In exercise, a beginner is a person who has decided to start an exercise routine or a person who has not worked out in the last twelve months. To progress from a beginner, be sure you have:

- Accurate information
- Precise directions

AMBIVALENT

An ambivalent exerciser has conflicting emotions and thoughts about whether it's worth the benefits or the effort it takes to workout. To overcome the feeling of ambiguity, be sure you:

- Use guilt to your advantage
- Consider working out with a partner
- Choose an exercise you enjoy

OBSESSIVE

An obsessive exerciser's effort is extreme. Your biggest challenge is to lessen your preoccupation. To move into balance, remember to:

- Keep perspective to prevent obsession

- Take time for yourself in ways other than exercising

BALANCED

A balanced exerciser understands that it's important to try for equilibrium in his or her life. As a balanced exerciser, you have learned moderation. You exercise and eat well, but not compulsively. You choose activities you enjoy and know you will pursue, so you don't need to feel guilty. You exercise with a partner if you want to, knowing a companion can make your exercise time more enjoyable. You stay informed, motivated and self-aware as much as possible, and that's enough. As a balanced exerciser, you are understanding:

- The importance of equilibrium within your life

- The importance of moderation in exercise and eating

- How to stay informed, motivated and self-aware

Your Personal Trainer has provided structure and the opportunity to challenge yourself, no matter what type you are.

Chapter Seven is the most challenging exercise routine so far. In order to stay motivated, you must give yourself the opportunity to persevere as you concentrate on the exercise. The accomplishment of finishing these exercises will benefit other parts of your life.

Chapter Seven is called cardiomuscular intensity because it works your muscular fibers deeply, developing them and reducing your intramuscular fat. Although you may feel you are able to do more than is asked each day, don't. More is not better.

NUTRITION

In Chapter Two the importance of eating healthy foods with the proper calorie intake was discussed. Watching what you eat, and eating wisely and carefully, will help you keep your energy level high as you exercise. We understand that there are times when it's difficult to eat regularly and during those times you may find yourself eating as an emotional response to a situation. Your awareness of this and your commitment to taking care of your body will help you make sound choices. It will also help you forgive yourself and continue when you fall short of your goals.

WHAT SHOULD YOU EAT?

Remember to eat a variety of foods each day, including fruits and vegetables, whole grain breads and cereals, lean meats, calcium rich foods, dry peas, beans, nuts and seeds.

If you're away from home, make small lunches and take them with you. Keep water with you during the day. Limit the amount of fat, saturated fat and cholesterol, including fat in meat, eggs, cream, butter or shortening.

Also, avoid eating too much sugar, including candy and soft drinks. The most important determining factor of what you eat will be how much you workout. If you pay attention, you'll notice that your body will tell you what healthy foods you should be eating.

MAKING CHOICES

Keeping a high energy level can be a challenge. So far we've talked about exercise and nutrition. What are the other factors that influence how you feel during the day? You must learn to choose your interactions and your activities carefully. For the sake of your health, difficult people and stressful situations MUST be avoided if possible. Learn to adapt to changes and modify your goals if necessary.
If you are confronted with a challenge, meet it, even if you're afraid. The questions you've been answering in the previous chapters may have already begun to increase your self-awareness. Continue this process, staying alert to the interactions of your physical and emotional self.

*Choose to do the best you can in each situation
as you imagine the best outcome.*

EXAMINING THE INFLUENCES TO MAKE BETTER CHOICES

Before you go to sleep tonight, think back over your day. Be aware of
the following:

> *Past experiences which are affecting you negatively now*

> *Past experiences which are affecting you positively now*

> *Present influences which are affecting you negatively now*

> *Present influences which are affecting you positively now*

> *Current goals which are most important to you and are
> affecting you positively now*

> *Current goals which are most important to you and are
> affecting you negatively now*

> *What actions you can take daily to rid yourself of the
> results of negative influences*

> *What actions you can take daily to reinforce the positive results
> of past and present influences.*

> *Which one or more of these influences you experience daily
> that made you feel enthusiastic and excited*

Answer these questions before you leave home:
How do you feel as you leave for school or work?

*Do you feel motivated and clear about what you want to accomplish
today? If not, what can you do to change this?*

Answer the following questions when you return home:
How did you feel during your day?

Did you plan all your activities for the day?   Yes   or   No
Were you able to stay with these plans?   Yes   or   No
If no, what happened?

What could you do next time to prevent this from happening?

Answer these questions at the end of your day:
How do you feel as the day is ending?

Did you accomplish what you wanted to accomplish?   Explain.

If you did, how can you reward yourself?

If you weren't able to reach your goals, what steps could you take
to help yourself come closer tomorrow?

In the morning there will be another written exercise to
start your day.

> **Just as you have created negative habits, you can create**
> **positive ones. You can learn to replace old responses with**
> **ones you choose.**

SCREENING FOR CANCER

Maintaining good overall health includes screening periodically for cancer and pre-cancer, because early detection can lead to a full cure in many cases. Not all cancers are detectable early, and not all can be screened for, but many can. We recommend the following cancer screening guidelines for early detection and/or prevention. If you're not familiar with any of these, ask your doctor for more information.

- For early prevention and detection of colon cancer, flexible sigmoidoscopy every three to five years in men and women 50 years and older. For people with a family history of colon cancer, start at age 40.

- For prevention and early detection of colon cancer, annual stool occult blood testing cards, beginning at age 50.

- For prevention and early detection of rectal cancer, for those with a family history of rectal cancer, have an annual rectal exam beginning at age 40.

- For early detection of prostate cancer, an annual prostate exam and PSA blood test in men 50 and over.

- For early detection of cervical cancer, an annual pap smear for women over 18 and/or those who have been sexually active.

- For detection of ovarian cancer, a pelvic exam every 1 to 3 years for women ages 18 to 40, and yearly for women over 40.

- For early detection of uterine cancer in women with a history of infertility, obesity, failure to ovulate, abnormal uterine bleeding, taking estrogen without progesterone or taking tamoxifen, an endometrial biopsy or a vaginal ultrasound.

- For early detection of breast cancer, a mammogram annually for women 40 and over.

- Monthly self-breast exam for women over 20.

- An office breast exam every three years for women ages 20 to 40, and annually after age 40.

A full medical exam, including health counseling and blood work, should be done as often as:

ages 20–30:	every 5 years
ages 30–40:	every 4 years
ages 40–50:	every 3 years
ages 50–60:	every 2 years

A good way to remember this is to have an exam two times in your 20's, three times in your 30's, four times in your 40's, five times in your 50's and yearly over 60.

ABOUT CANCER
The kinds, the risks, early detection and prevention

LUNG CANCER
Lung cancer is the second most common cause of death in the United States. It causes 25% of cancer deaths. For a smoker who smokes two packs a day for twenty years, the risk of lung cancer is about seventy times greater than for a nonsmoker. Once a smoker quits smoking, it takes about fifteen years for his or her risk of cancer to return to that of the general population.

Screening for lung cancer: Unfortunately, there's no good tool for early detection of lung cancer. Yearly chest x-rays and sputum cytologies aren't recommended, as they pick up cancer too late to do any good. The best solution for preventing lung cancer is to not smoke. The death rate is decreasing in Caucasian males due to lower smoking rates in this group. However, it continues to increase in women and African-American males as their smoking rates have risen.

COLON CANCER
There's a 6% lifetime risk of developing colon cancer. The risk increases to approximately 12 to 18% if anyone in the immediate family has a history of it. Also at increased risk are people with multiple recurring colon polyps, people with previous colon cancer or adenomatous polyps, a history of ulcerative colitis for more than 7 years or a history of female genital cancer.

Screening for colon cancer: For everyone, minimum screening will help detect polyps that may turn into colon cancer. This should include flexible sigmoidoscopy every three years and yearly stool occult blood testing after age 50. At a minimum, high risk patients should have colonoscopy or flexible sigmoidoscopy with a barium enema every three to five years, along with yearly occult blood testing starting at age 40.

BREAST CANCER

A woman living to age 85 has a one in ten chance of having breast cancer at some time in her life. The risk increases with each decade of life. In the United States, the median age for breast cancer is 58. Therefore, while breast self-exam, physician exam and mammogram is important before age fifty, they become increasingly important after that. For instance, the chances of a mammogram finding breast cancer is much higher in a 70 year old woman than a 40 year old woman. Blood tests, ultrasound and thermography are of no value in routine screening. One way to reduce the risk of breast cancer is for women to breast-feed their babies a minimum of three months for each baby. Each succeeding baby reduces the risk even more.

Breast cancer risk is affected by family history. Studies on this have produced varying reports, but an average risk can be given. In general, a woman's risk increases by 2 to 2.5 times if her mother had breast cancer between the ages 40 and 70, and by 1.5 if her mother had breast cancer after 70 years old.

Screening: all women should learn self-exam techniques and do these monthly. A yearly physician exam is important. Starting at 40 years old, all women should have a yearly mammogram.

The following table lists risk of having had breast cancer by age group:

Age	Odds
25	1 in 19,606
30	1 in 2,525
35	1 in 606
40	1 in 217

45	1 in	93
50	1 in	50
55	1 in	33
60	1 in	24
65	1 in	17
70	1 in	14
75	1 in	11
80	1 in	10
85	1 in	9
95 or older	1 in	8

USN&WR - Data: National Cancer Institute.

PROSTATE CANCER

Prostate cancer is generally considered a disease of the elderly, rarely occurring before age 50 and reaching its peak by the time men are in their 70's. Although a Prostate Specific Antigen (PSA) will be abnormal in 5 to 6% of men over 50, only 30 to 40% of these men will actually be found to have cancer. Early detection of prostate cancer relies on the digital rectal exam and the PSA for men over age 50. If either is abnormal, a prostatic ultrasound and free PSA can be done to help determine if cancer is present. When prostate cancer is detected while it's still localized within the prostate, it can be considered fully curable. But prostate cancer which has spread beyond the prostate isn't curable. Thus, early detection of this cancer is important. Despite these factors routine PSA testing remains controversial, because PSA's are not exact and can be misleading.

CERVICAL CANCER

Cervical cancer is now considered a sexually transmitted disease, spread by contact with certain wart viruses, called human papilloma virus. The virus may be unknowingly contracted and then remain present for years. Eventually, it can cause cell changes in the cervix which can lead to cervical cancer. The best screening technique is the pap smear, which detects any changes years before they cause cancer. Because the virus may remain present without causing immediate change, it's important to have regular pap smears.

OVARIAN CANCER

Ovarian cancer occurs in approximately 1.4% of women, usually after menopause. There is a much greater risk if a mother, sister or daughter has a history of ovarian cancer, and this risk increases even more with two relatives. The blood test, CA-125, is inadequate at predicting ovarian cancer and shouldn't be used for screening. Ultrasound is controversial and shouldn't be used routinely, but it may be helpful for women who are at risk because of family history. After menopause and childbearing, removal of the ovaries is recommended for women with a strong family history of ovarian cancer.

UTERINE CANCER

Women who take estrogen without progesterone are at an increased risk for uterine cancer. The risk also increases for women with a history of infertility, irregular bleeding, obesity, failure to ovulate and the use of tamoxifen after breast cancer. A routine pap smear doesn't screen well for this type of cancer. A pelvic exam can be helpful, but it isn't completely adequate. The best screening techniques include endometrial biopsy and vaginal probe ultrasound.

MELANOMA

Melanoma is increasingly becoming a cause of skin cancer in the United States. In certain parts of Australia the risk of melanoma is as high as 30-40%. It's also the one skin cancer that can commonly cause death by metastasis and can even affect the younger age groups. Because melanoma starts as a dysplastic nevus (an atypical mole), it's important to stay aware of any moles you may have. A particularly suspicious mole is one that's growing or changing rapidly, is blackening or developing a blue or red pigmentation, is becoming irregular along the borders or is developing an irregular area somewhere within the mole itself.

Doctors use the A, B, C, D's to look for potentially dangerous moles.
A is for asymmetry
B is for border irregularity
C is for color changes (red, blue or black within a mole)
D is for dimension greater than 6 millimeters
(the diameter of a pencil's eraser)

If you have any questions about moles you have, check them with your health care provider. Like ovarian cancer, the risk of melanoma increases with family history. The presence of a dysplastic nevus plus a family history of melanoma increases the chances of melanoma 148 times. Presence of an atypical pigmented lesion or atypical mole, but without the family history, gives an increased risk of 70 times the normal risk.

To decrease the risk of melanoma, have routine exams, wear a hat and shirt and at least SPF 15 sun block when outside, and avoid prolonged exposure to the sun between 10 a.m. and 2 p.m., even with protection. If you have moles, see your doctor for an exam and learn to do self-exams. Questionable moles can be biopsied or photographed for observation over time.

WORKOUT: CARDIOMUSCULAR INTENSITY
LOWER BODY ROUTINE

Cardiomuscular intensity provides deep muscular fiber strengthening and toning. Because of this, it may feel like the most difficult. But remember, you have prepared yourself for this type of workout. Just keep in mind that you are to:

- Focus on the part of the body you are exercising

- Visualize each movement before you perform it

- Imagine what your body will look like because you are exercising

- Stay aware of the changes you have made

- Control your exercise so you don't work too hard or too little

How do you feel before starting your workout?

☐ Motivated ☐ Discouraged

☐ Excited ☐ Dreading

☐ Pressed for time ☐ Resigned

☐ Confident ☐ Anxious

☐ Not sure ☐ Ready and willing

☐ Clear-minded ☐ Don't want to think about it

Do you know why you're doing this. Yes No Explain:

How do these answers compare to your previous ones?
Is there a difference? Why?

W A L K / J O G OR B I K E

Time _____ *HR* _____		*Time* _____ *HR* _____	
Start _____		*Start* _____	
@ 6 min	_____	@ 6 min	_____
@12 min	_____	@ 12 min	_____
@18 min	_____	@ 18 min	_____
@20 min	_____	@ 20 min	_____
Stop _____		*Stop* _____	

Don't rest when you have finished with the cardiovascular part of the workout. This next set of exercises may feel like the most difficult ones you have performed but it's important to persevere with confidence. Don't rest between reps.

The first set will be the most difficult, because your body will be adjusting to doing the exercise. Continue exercising, checking to make sure you maintain correct positions, especially during the first five reps. During the 5th through 9th reps your body will have adjusted and the movements will feel more comfortable. But as you continue, during the 10th through 16th reps, you may feel out of breath and your muscles may start to feel a burning sensation.

13 through 18 reps are the pain threshold to get through. If you can continue through distractions and discomfort, you'll find yourself adapting both physically and mentally. Give yourself a chance to find this part of yourself and the effects will spread to all parts of your life. Continue to exercise carefully and with concentration. To help you get through this period, take slow and controlled breaths. When you reach the 17th through 20th reps, you may experience a sensation of fullness in the areas you're working.

Try to keep exercising. It's normal to feel like stopping to rest, but continue if you can. Some of the reasons for wanting to stop are:

■ You feel a burning sensation

■ Someone interrupts your concentration

■ You have past painful or negative experiences, which make you feel you can't persevere

LOWER BODY ROUTINE
1. Leg squats - 2 sets of 20 reps with no weight
Rest for 30 seconds after the first and second set and check your heart rate after the second set: _____

2. Walking Lunges - 2 sets of 20 reps each leg with no weight
Rest for 30 seconds after the first and second set and check your heart rate after the second set: _____

3. *Adductor (inner thighs) - 2 sets of 20 reps*
Small builds use 5 – 20 lbs if using leg pulley or ankle weights or use
20 – 50 lbs if using an adductor machine
Large builds use 10 – 20 lbs if using leg pulley or ankle weights or use
40 – 80 lbs if using an adductor machine
Rest for 30 seconds after the first and second set

5. Standing Alternating Leg Curls or Lying Leg Curls -
2 sets of 20 reps
Smaller builds use 10 - 20 lbs of ankle weights or 20 - 40 lbs
Larger builds use 20 - 30 lbs of ankle weights or 40 - 70 lbs
Rest for 30 seconds after the first and second set

6. Seated Leg Extension - 2 sets of 20 reps
Smaller builds use 20 lbs of ankle weights or on a machine
use 20 - 40 lbs
Larger builds use 30 lbs of ankle weights or on a machine
use 40 - 70 lbs
Rest for 30 seconds after the first and second set and check
your heart rate after the second set: _____

7.   *Standing One Leg Calf Raises - 2 sets of 20 reps, with no weights*

8.   *Flat Back Leg Raises - 2 sets of 50 reps with no weights*

9.   *Flat Back Crunch Ups - 2 sets of 50 reps with no weight,*
     Don't rest between reps

10. *Side Crunch Ups - 2 sets of 50 reps with no weight,*
     Don't rest between reps

11. *Flat Stomach Back Raises - 2 sets of 50 reps with no weight*
     Don't rest between reps

Complete today's session by doing your stretching exercise

How did you feel during your workout?

☐ I needed more energy ☐ I had too many negative thoughts

☐ I could have gone on forever ☐ I felt good after it was over

☐ I like how I'm feeling ☐ I need a partner

☐ I just wasn't interested today ☐ I felt powerful

☐ What an invigorating feeling ☐ It's good to have my body active

Were you able to keep yourself motivated?
If so, how?
If not, why not?

How do you feel now that your workout is finished?

☐ Glad it's over ☐ Joyful

☐ Feel good about what I accomplished ☐ Poised

☐ Can't wait until next time ☐ Gratified

☐ I wish I'd started this long ago ☐ Rejuvenated

☐ Now I understand why this is important ☐ Successful

I think and feel I am on my way to becoming more fit.
Yes   No   Explain:

Trainer's Comments & Suggestions:

Your daily routine will make the difference between success and failure. If you know how you are spending your time each day, you can increase your chance of success.
How are your actual times comparing to your goal times?

THYROID & WEIGHT GAIN

Patients frequently ask their doctors if their weight problem or recent weight gain is caused by low thyroid. In most cases, thyroid isn't the cause. But if this is a concern, simple TSH (thyroid stimulating hormone) and T4 blood tests can give you the answer. The classic symptoms of low thyroid are weight gain, coarse skin, fatigue, sluggish reflexes, depression and constipation. However, many people have one or even all of these symptoms and don't have hypothyroidism. Since thyroid supplementation in patients with normal TSH increases the risk of health problems, especially osteoporosis, don't take thyroid medication unless your blood tests indicate low thyroid levels.

DIABETES . . .

is defined as two consecutive fasting blood sugars of 125 mg./Dl or more. Symptoms include excessive urination, frequent nighttime urination, extreme thirst and greatly increased appetite. Although diabetes can be hereditary, in adults it's also linked to being overweight and underactive. Uncontrolled diabetes can triple the risk of stroke and heart attack. It can also cause blindness, kidney failure, skin infections, loss of limbs and other complications.

There are two types of diabetes. Type 1 usually starts in childhood and is due to the destruction of the pancreas which results in no insulin production. In Type 2, the adult and most common type of diabetes, the pancreas makes extra insulin but the insulin doesn't work well. There is "insulin resistance." The body's cells don't absorb sugar from the blood and also the liver pumps out too much sugar. Diabetes increases the risk of heart disease, especially in women, by laying down more plaque in the coronary arteries.

DAY 44　　TODAY'S DATE:
The following questions can help keep you aware of how you are approaching your day. Think about them each day.

How did you feel when you wake up?

Did you get enough sleep?　　If no, why not?

How did your dreams make you feel about yourself?

If a dream or event affected you negatively, what do you need to work on to help you think more positively about yourself?

When you think about these questions before you leave home, they can help prepare you for your day.
How do you feel as you leave for school or work?

Do you feel motivated and clear about what you want to accomplish? If not, what can you do to change this?

When you think about these questions after you return, they can help you begin to unwind from the day.
How did you feel during your day?

Did you plan all your activities for the day?

Were you able to stay with these plans?

If no, what happened? What could you do next time to prevent this from happening?

When you think about these questions at the end of the day, they can help you begin to redirect your efforts in a positive direction.

How do you feel as the day is ending?

Did you accomplish what you wanted to accomplish?

If you did, how can you reward yourself?

If you weren't able to reach your goals, what steps can you take to help yourself come closer?

Workout: Cardiomuscular Intensity
Upper Body Routine

How do you feel before starting your workout?
Why are you doing this.
How do these thoughts compare to your previous ones?
Is there a difference?   Why?

ROW		WALK/JOG OR BIKE	
Time _____ *HR* _____		*Time* _____ *HR* _____	
*Start*_____		*Start*_____	
@ 6 min	_____	@ 6 min	_____
@12 min	_____	@ 12 min	_____
@18 min	_____	@ 18 min	_____
@20 min	_____	@ 20 min	_____
*Stop*_____		*Stop* _____	

Make sure to drink plenty of water.

While you're performing the next group of exercises, you may feel increased tightness and a strong burning sensation. At times you may also feel out of breath and your shoulders may ache. As you did for your lower body, try to continue exercising without resting between repetitions. Again, it's important to maintain proper alignment. Watch for this during the first five reps.

During the first twelve reps, the muscles will start to produce waste products in the form of lactic acid. As the exercises become more difficult, take slow and controlled breaths. Between reps 5 and 9, your arms may begin to feel tight. Between reps 13 and 16, they may begin to burn and hurt, and between 17 and 20, your arms, shoulders and back may start to burn. Your breathing may also become labored. Continue exercising if you can and your body will adjust. Again, when your heart rate is at this level, you may find excuses for stopping. These can include:

- You have a burning sensation

- Someone interrupts your concentration

- You have past painful and negative experiences, making you feel you can't persevere

Continue, if you can. Remember 13 and 18 reps are the pain threshold for positive benefits. If you can continue through distractions and discomfort, you'll find yourself adapting both mentally and physically. Give yourself a chance to find this part of yourself and the effects will spread to all parts of your life. Continue to exercise carefully and with concentration. You should find the second set to be much easier than the first, because your body has adjusted. You may feel more energetic and able to respond to the demands of the exercises.

UPPER BODY ROUTINE

1. Seated Lat Rows 2 sets of 20 reps
Smaller builds use 20 to 60 lbs
Larger builds use 50 to 100 lbs
Rest for 30 seconds and check your heart rate after the first set: _____

2. Push-ups or Chest Press- 2 sets of 20 reps
Smaller builds use 20 to 40 lbs
Larger builds use 40 to 100 lbs
Rest for 30 seconds after the first set and check your heart rate after the second set: _____

3. Lat Pull Downs - 2 sets of 20 reps
Smaller builds use 20 to 40 lbs
Larger builds use 50 to 110 lbs
Rest for 30 seconds after the first and second set

4. Flat Bench Chest Flies - 2 sets of 20 reps
Smaller builds use 3 to 10 lbs
Larger builds use 10 to 60 lbs
Rest for 30 seconds after the first and second set

5. Side Lateral Raises - 2 sets of 20 reps, with dumbbells
Smaller builds use 3 to 10 lbs
Larger builds use 15 to 25 lbs
Rest for 30 seconds after the first and second set

6. Triceps Kick Backs - 2 sets of 20 reps
Smaller builds use 10 to 20 lbs
Larger builds use 30 to 50 lbs
Rest for 30 seconds after the second set

7. One Arm Biceps Curls - 2 sets of 20 reps, using dumbbells
Smaller builds use 5 to 15 lbs
Larger builds use 20 to 40 lbs
Rest for 30 seconds after the and second set

8. Forearm Curls / 2 sets of 20 reps
Smaller builds use 10 - 20 lbs
Larger builds use 20 - 40 lbs
Rest for 30 seconds after the first set

9. Flat Back Leg Raises–2 sets of 50 reps

10. Flat Back Crunch Ups–2 sets of 50 reps

11. Side Crunches–2 sets of 50 reps

12. Flat Stomach Back Raises–2 sets of 50 reps

When you've finished, perform your stretching exercises.
Hold each position for a 30 second.

Keep in mind:

How you felt during your workout.

How you were able to keep yourself motivated.

How you felt after you finished.

Trainer's Comments & Suggestions:

FIBROMYALGIA . . .
is a pain disorder. The symptoms of fibromyalgia include body aches, joint aches, fatigue, headache and painful trigger points. Not much is known about this disease, including how common it actually is.

It's classified as a connective tissue disorder, along with more well-known diseases, such as rheumatoid arthritis and lupus. Fibromyalgia may also include some kind of sleep disorder. So far, there are no good tests to diagnose it and the cause of it is unknown. Exercise, from light to moderate, has been found to be helpful in treating fibromyalgia, as well as some medications in the antidepressant family.

CHRONIC PAIN
Do you have it? Many people have pain, either from an old injury to the back, neck, arm or leg, or from arthritis, fibromyalgia or tension headaches. When all standard acute treatments don't cure the problem, and pain becomes chronic, a simple standard chronic pain treatment regimen will help. The first and more important step in treatment is regular exercise, such as described in this book. Second, if pain is severe, then specific nonsteroidal, anti-inflammatory medication taken either regularly or intermittently will help. Acetaminophen may be helpful, as well. Surprisingly, taking ongoing antidepressant medication can significantly reduce pain. These medications block pain receptors in the brain, lessening one's ability to sense pain.

EXERCISE AFTER INJURY
If you sustain an injury and you're in good shape, should you keep exercising? Yes, if possible, so you don't lose your cardiovascular fitness.
Often you can find an alternative exercise that doesn't stress the injured area. Swimming and stationary bicycling are often excellent choices. If you have a lower extremity injury, you can often find exercises to work your upper extremities and vice versa.

DAY 45   TODAY'S DATE:
A DAY FOR MASSAGE, MEDITATION AND SILENCE

Although today is a day off from physical exercise, make sure you are paying attention to your nutritional intake. Continue to give yourself 30 minutes for your meditation time. During this time for silence you will concentrate on visualizing your favorite place of retreat. When you close your eyes, think of a place that feels peaceful. Now follow the directions for meditation I or II.

If possible, arrange to have a full body massage today or tomorrow. Having a massage will help to relax you and heal any muscular pains you may have. You may feel as if massages are a luxury; don't, they have important physical and mental benefits.

Let's look at your time goals again.
How do your actual times compare to your goal time routine?

    1. What time do you want to wake up?

        Goal time_____   Actual time_____

    2. What time do you want to get out of bed?

        Goal time_____   Actual time_____

    3. How long will it take you to eat your first meal?

        Goal time_____   Actual time_____

    4. What time will you leave for work/school/other?

        Goal time_____   Actual time_____

    5. What time will you arrive at work?

        Goal time_____   Actual time_____

    6. What time will you start work?

        Goal time_____   Actual time_____

    7. How long will it take you to eat your first snack?

        Goal time_____   Actual time_____

8. After you finish your snack, when will you work?

Goal time_____   Actual time_____

9. How long will your break be?

Goal time_____   Actual time_____

10. How long will it take you to eat your lunch?

Goal time_____   Actual time_____

11. What time will you work after you finish your lunch?

Goal time_____   Actual time_____

12. How long will it take you to eat your second snack?

Goal time_____   Actual time_____

13. What time will you leave work?

Goal time_____   Actual time_____

14. How long will it take you to get home?

Goal time_____   Actual time_____

15. What time will you have your dinner?

Goal time_____   Actual time_____

16. How much time will you spend watching television?

Goal time_____   Actual time_____

17. How much time will you take for personal quiet time?

Goal time_____   Actual time_____

18. How much time will you spend exercising?

Goal time_____   Actual time_____

19. How much time will you devote to family time?

Goal time_____   Actual time_____

20. How much time will you devote to work study?

Goal time_____   Actual time_____

21. How much time will you spend in pleasure reading?

Goal time_____   Actual time_____

22. How much time will you spend school studying?

Goal time_____   Actual time_____

23. How much time will you spend socializing with friends?

Goal time_____   Actual time_____

24. How much time will you devote to chores?

Goal time_____   Actual time_____

25. What time will you go to bed?

Goal time_____   Actual time_____

LIPOSUCTION

Have you exercised down to your ideal weight and still have excessive fat in some places? Certain areas of fat distribution, such as saddlebags (bulges in upper, outer thigh), love handles (fat at the iliac crest), and fat in the lower abdomen can be resistant to exercise. This fat may remain even after exercising, modifying your food intake and reaching the ideal weight.

Acceptable methods to get rid of these 'leftovers' include liposuction and tummy tucks. Check on these procedures, only after getting down to your ideal weight, and only if you don't smoke. Make sure that you research a reputable doctor for these procedures. For women: fat above the umbilicus is usually taken off easily. However, fat below the umbilicus is more resistant to proper nutrition and exercise, especially if you have had a C-section.

DAY 46   TODAY'S DATE:
WORKOUT: CARDIOMUSCULAR INTENSITY
LOWER BODY ROUTINE

WALK/JOG   OR   BIKE

WALK/JOG		BIKE	
Time _____ HR _____		*Time* _____ HR _____	
Start _____		*Start* _____	
@ 6 min	_____	@ 6 min	_____
@ 12 min	_____	@ 12 min	_____
@ 18 min	_____	@ 18 min	_____
@ 20 min	_____	@ 20 min	_____
Stop _____		*Stop* _____	

Make sure you are drinking plenty of water.

Follow lower body routine for Day 43. (pages, 11-15). When you finished, perform your stretching exercises. Do each for 30 seconds.

Trainer's Comments & Suggestions:

HEART DISEASE
Is there a strong history of heart disease in your family? If so, ask your doctor to check your blood homocysteine levels. If your level is high, you can undergo further testing to confirm hyperhomocysteinemia. If you find out you have it, you can dramatically decrease your risk of heart disease by taking folic acid, 1 mg./day. Folic acid counteracts the damage this genetic disorder does to the heart.

In general, women are at lower risk of heart attack and coronary disease than men of the same age. Premenopausal women tend to be at particularly low risk. With coronary risk, women tend to lag 10 years behind men. But risk increases progressively after menopause, eventually more closely paralleling the risk of men. The use of estrogen after menopause for women helps negate a woman's risk.

DAY 47   TODAY'S DATE:
CARDIOMUSCULAR INTENSITY - UPPER BODY ROUTINE

R O W   W A L K / J O G   OR   B I K E

Time _____ *HR* _____		*Time* _____ *HR* _____	
Start _____		*Start* _____	
@ 6 min	_____	@ 6 min	_____
@12 min	_____	@ 12 min	_____
@18 min	_____	@ 18 min	_____
@20 min	_____	@ 20 min	_____
Stop _____		*Stop* _____	

Make sure to drink plenty of water.

Rest for 60 seconds before starting the next exercises

Follow the upper body routine for Day 44 (pages, 17-21).
When you've finished, perform your stretching exercises.
Hold each position for a 30 second count.

Trainer's Comments & Suggestions:

It's important to keep track of your time.
How are your actual times comparing with your goal times?
Are they starting to come closer?

DAY 48   TODAY'S DATE:
STAYING MOTIVATED AND AWARE OF HOW YOU FEEL
At times, it can seem overwhelming to stay motivated and aware of
how you think and feel during the day. *Your Personal Trainer* allows
you to have insight into the impact your daily events have on your
moods and attitudes. In order to move from being a beginner through
ambivalence or obsessiveness to balance, it's important that you
examine as many influences as you can. This will help you change
your perspective and give you more control over your reactions to
events that make you unbalanced. You can't always control what
happens to you in your life, but you can learn to control your reactions
and the effect your reactions have on you. An important ingredient in
this process is making sure that you examine the influences that determine your actions.

EXAMINING THE INFLUENCES IN YOUR DAILY LIFE
Before you go to sleep tonight, think back over your day.
Can you recall moments that changed your thinking or feeling?
Did these events cause your energy to increase or lessen?

List the following:

Past experiences which are affecting you negatively now:

Past experiences which are affecting you positively now:

Present influences which are affecting you negatively now:

Present influences which are affecting you positively now:

*Current goals which are most important to you and are affecting
you positively now:*

Current goals which are most important to you and are affecting you negatively now:

List the actions you took today to rid yourself of the results of the negative influences:

List the actions you took today to reinforce the positive results of past and present influences:

Past:

Present

List one or more of these influences you experienced today that made you feel enthusiastic and excited:

When you've finished this exercise, have a good night's sleep.

In the morning there will be another written exercise to start your day. The following exercise will help you start your day more aware of how you are approaching your day.

Answer these questions before you get out of bed in the morning:
How did you feel when you woke up?

Did you get enough sleep?   *Yes*   *No*
If no, why not?

How did your dreams make you feel about yourself?

If a dream or event affected you negatively, what do you need to work on today to help you think more positively about yourself?

Answer these questions before you leave home:
How do you feel as you leave for school or work?

Do you feel motivated and clear about what you want to accomplish today? If not, what can you do to change this?

Answer these questions when you return home:
How did you feel during your day?

Did you plan all your activities for the day?	*Yes*	*or*	*No*
Were you able to stay with these plans?	*Yes*	*or*	*No*
If no, what happened?			

What could you do next time to prevent this from happening?

Answer these questions at the end of your day:
How do you feel as the day is ending?
Did you accomplish what you wanted to accomplish? Explain.

If you did, how can you reward yourself?

If you weren't able to reach your goals, what can be done to help you come closer tomorrow?

Your Personal Trainer's approach to taking more control over your life is to repeat positive behaviors over and over. However, to ensure that these behaviors are maintained, it's important that you exercise. Remember, if negative behaviors can be maintained, so can positive ones. As you learn to examine your daily life, including your expectations and your accomplishments, you will see how you can change unwanted patterns.

MENOPAUSE, ESTROGEN & EXERCISE FOR WOMEN

Women can help prevent two major causes of injury, illness and death after menopause by exercising and taking estrogen after menopause. There is now clear-cut evidence that both aerobic exercise and estrogen post-menopause significantly reduce the risk of coronary artery disease in women. The effect of estrogen may be great enough to negate elevated cholesterol.

Osteoporosis (and subsequent hip fractures in elderly women) is a far too common cause of major disability and often eventual death. The addition of estrogen starting at menopause, along with weight bearing exercise throughout life, play a major role in reducing the risk of osteoporosis. Estrogen has some drawbacks, but should be discussed at length with a woman's physician as menopause approaches.

DAY 49 TODAY'S DATE:
I'M LEARNING TO THINK AND FEEL IN A NEW WAY

At this point in, you have been taught skills that can help you change many of your old negative habits. These skills will help you cope with the many obstacles you may have encountered in the past as you tried to change your lifestyle patterns.

How to overcome the normal resistance to new thinking:

You may have tried other lifestyle change routines or exercise routines and eventually given up. Or, you may have reached a particular goal and then stopped, eventually finding yourself back where you started. *Your Personal Trainer* has provided you with techniques that will help you learn how to have confidence in your ability to achieve physical and mental fitness by reaching the goals you set for yourself. This will also help you to make a healthy lifestyle a permanent part of your life.

You have learned how to:

- Believe in yourself and the techniques you are using

- Persist even when change is slow

- Take care of yourself

- Think independently

- Use exercise to help you stay motivated

Change is difficult for everyone. Developing new habits, then feeling comfortable with them is an essential part of the adjustment. This book helps provide motivation through transition. Our emphasis is on consistency and repetition, so that your body and mind have a chance to learn new behaviors and replace old ones.

You have gained new skills in how to recognize and overcome thoughts which have hindered you in the past. It's natural to feel overwhelmed or unsure with a new approach to life.

NEW MOTIVATION

There may have been times in your life when you have felt the effort to do anything was too much. Now you may have more control of your concentration, sleep disturbances, headaches or back pains. You are learning you can cope with these feelings without having to start or increase the use of food, alcohol or drugs. You may also find that you don't have to alternate between feeling positive about yourself and feeling anxious, maybe even phobic. As you use this book, your list of shoulds' can become a list of wills'.

What is happening to create this new attitude?

Through exercise, writing, meditation and information, you are learning to recognize the negative and positive influences in your life. You are learning to choose change as a way to feel better about yourself. And, most importantly, you are aware that this change isn't a short-term solution but an ongoing process.

CHAPTER EIGHT

STAY HEALTHY AND FIT AS A WAY OF LIFE

NOTICE HOW YOU'VE CHANGED
LOOK AT WHAT YOU'VE ACCOMPLISHED
KEEP PERSPECTIVE IN YOUR LIFE
REFLECT ON WHAT YOU'VE LEARNED ABOUT YOURSELF

DAY 50   TODAY'S DATE:
NOTICE HOW YOU'VE CHANGED

To maintain a healthier way of life it is important to understand the stages you went through to reach this point. Each chapter in this book has taken you further along with your exercise, your knowledge, your nutrition and your self-awareness.

That is our goal: to educate you, both physically and mentally. By using incremental steps, you've been able to achieve more than you may have thought you could. It's easy to feel overwhelmed when you're only able to see the contrast between where you are and where you want to be. Learning to set a goal, using patience and determination to move toward it, and observing yourself in the process is important to any lifestyle change. You have done all of these in the past weeks. Your reward for this isn't just increased fitness, it's also the knowledge that you have the ability to persevere. We hope this knowledge will be applied to other parts of your life.

As you may remember, we discussed your negative and positive energy levels. Answer the 50 questions and you will be able to look again at how you're affected by various influences in your life. Read each question and put a check by the most appropriate response.

1. *I have lots of energy and I look forward to each day.*
   ☐ Never ☐ Seldom ☐ Sometimes ☐ Often ☐ Always

2. *I find a challenge exciting.*
   ☐ Never ☐ Seldom ☐ Sometimes ☐ Often ☐ Always

3. *I show good judgment when I experience a difficult situation.*
   ☐ Never ☐ Seldom ☐ Sometimes ☐ Often ☐ Always

4. *When I feel rushed and have deadlines to meet, I think of them as challenges.*
   ☐ Never ☐ Seldom ☐ Sometimes ☐ Often ☐ Always

5. *I believe that if I persist, I will overcome adversity.*
   ☐ Never ☐ Seldom ☐ Sometimes ☐ Often ☐ Always

6. *To avoid feeling overwhelmed, I set mental and physical goals that are attainable.*
   ☐ Never ☐ Seldom ☐ Sometimes ☐ Often ☐ Always

7. *I believe in my ability to remain faithful to my values.*
   ☐ Never ☐ Seldom ☐ Sometimes ☐ Often ☐ Always

8. *I feel motivated and determined.*
   ☐ Never ☐ Seldom ☐ Sometimes ☐ Often ☐ Always

9. *I can maintain my concentration to achieve a goal.*
   ☐ Never ☐ Seldom ☐ Sometimes ☐ Often ☐ Always

10. *To accomplish my goals, I keep myself ready and alert.*
    ☐ Never ☐ Seldom ☐ Sometimes ☐ Often ☐ Always

11.   I am happy with the decisions I make.
☐ Never   ☐ Seldom   ☐ Sometimes   ☐ Often   ☐ Always

12.   When I feel stressed or depressed, I use exercise to relieve my feelings.
☐ Never   ☐ Seldom   ☐ Sometimes   ☐ Often   ☐ Always

13.   When I feel overwhelmed or fatigued, I use a brief period of relaxation to rejuvenate myself.
☐ Never   ☐ Seldom   ☐ Sometimes   ☐ Often   ☐ Always

14.   I eat a balanced intake of food.
☐ Never   ☐ Seldom   ☐ Sometimes   ☐ Often   ☐ Always

15.   I take regular vacations.
☐ Never   ☐ Seldom   ☐ Sometimes   ☐ Often   ☐ Always

16.   I enjoy interacting with others.
☐ Never   ☐ Seldom   ☐ Sometimes   ☐ Often   ☐ Always

17.   I am able to achieve goals I have set for myself.
☐ Never   ☐ Seldom   ☐ Sometimes   ☐ Often   ☐ Always

18.   I have the support I need.
☐ Never   ☐ Seldom   ☐ Sometimes   ☐ Often   ☐ Always

19.   I use incentives to keep me focused on my goals.
☐ Never   ☐ Seldom   ☐ Sometimes   ☐ Often   ☐ Always

20.   When I want to make changes in my life, I ask for help.
☐ Never   ☐ Seldom   ☐ Sometimes   ☐ Often   ☐ Always

21. *I am happy with the choices I have made so far in my life.*
☐ Never ☐ Seldom ☐ Sometimes ☐ Often ☐ Always

22. *I stay motivated so I can accomplish my goals.*
☐ Never ☐ Seldom ☐ Sometimes ☐ Often ☐ Always

23. *I have the incentive, the knowledge and the support to change any unhealthy behaviors.*
☐ Never ☐ Seldom ☐ Sometimes ☐ Often ☐ Always

24. *I act contrary to my common sense and wants.*
☐ Never ☐ Seldom ☐ Sometimes ☐ Often ☐ Always

25. *I feel tired for no apparent reason.*
☐ Never ☐ Seldom ☐ Sometimes ☐ Often ☐ Always

26. *I feel confused and helpless.*
☐ Never ☐ Seldom ☐ Sometimes ☐ Often ☐ Always

27. *Because I feel uneasy around others, I avoid socializing*
☐ Never ☐ Seldom ☐ Sometimes ☐ Often ☐ Always

28. *I have fears which prevent me from acting decisively.*
☐ Never ☐ Seldom ☐ Sometimes ☐ Often ☐ Always

29. *Other people can make me feel rushed, stressed or worried.*

☐ Never ☐ Seldom ☐ Sometimes ☐ Often ☐ Always

30. *There are times when I don't have the courage to act decisively.*
☐ Never ☐ Seldom ☐ Sometimes ☐ Often ☐ Always

31.   *I feel restless and edgy.*
☐ Never   ☐ Seldom   ☐ Sometimes   ☐ Often   ☐ Always

33.   *I have strong fears of situations I'm powerless to control or avoid.*
☐ Never   ☐ Seldom   ☐ Sometimes   ☐ Often   ☐ Always

35.   *I feel I've reached a point where I need to make changes, but I'm not motivated.*
☐ Never   ☐ Seldom   ☐ Sometimes   ☐ Often   ☐ Always

36.   *I have bowel problems - constipation, diarrhea, pain or bloating.*
☐ Never   ☐ Seldom   ☐ Sometimes   ☐ Often   ☐ Always

37.   *I have brief periods of excessive agitation.*
☐ Never   ☐ Seldom   ☐ Sometimes   ☐ Often   ☐ Always

38.   *I have difficulty functioning as I have in the past.*
☐ Never   ☐ Seldom   ☐ Sometimes   ☐ Often   ☐ Always

39.   *When I feel frustrated with my life, I don't want to face others. I would rather stay home to avoid any contact.*
☐ Never   ☐ Seldom   ☐ Sometimes   ☐ Often   ☐ Always

40.   *I feel depressed.*
☐ Never   ☐ Seldom   ☐ Sometimes   ☐ Often   ☐ Always

41.   *I find myself overeating when I feel stressed or depressed.*
☐ Never   ☐ Seldom   ☐ Sometimes   ☐ Often   ☐ Always

42.   *I have a decreased sex drive.*
☐ Never   ☐ Seldom   ☐ Sometimes   ☐ Often   ☐ Always

43.   *I find it hard to concentrate or feel motivated When I feel like this, I move too slowly to accomplish anything.*
☐ Never   ☐ Seldom   ☐ Sometimes   ☐ Often   ☐ Always

44.   *I have trouble getting the same pleasure from my life I once got.*
☐ Never   ☐ Seldom   ☐ Sometimes   ☐ Often   ☐ Always

45.   *I use alcohol or drugs as a means of relaxation.*
☐ Never   ☐ Seldom   ☐ Sometimes   ☐ Often   ☐ Always

46.   *I have thoughts of harming myself or committing suicide.*
☐ Never   ☐ Seldom   ☐ Sometimes   ☐ Often   ☐ Always

47.   *I feel inadequate.*
☐ Never   ☐ Seldom   ☐ Sometimes   ☐ Often   ☐ Always

48.   *I wish I had taken a different direction earlier in life.*
☐ Never   ☐ Seldom   ☐ Sometimes   ☐ Often   ☐ Always

49.   *I don't have enough time for myself, my family or my friends.*
☐ Never   ☐ Seldom   ☐ Sometimes   ☐ Often   ☐ Always

50.   *I have verbal disagreements with others.*
☐ Never   ☐ Seldom   ☐ Sometimes   ☐ Often   ☐ Always

Now add up the points for the questions in Chapter Eight and place the totals here.

Points for questions 1 – 23   +_____

Points for questions 24 – 50   - _____

Take the positive and negative scores from:
Chapter One and place the total here +
Chapter One and place the total here -
Chapter Four and place the total here +
Chapter Four and place the total here -

Using the following graph, plot your six scores. You will be comparing your + (positive) scores and your - (negative) scores. Under Chapters One, Four and Eight, place your (+) score above the line and your (-) score below the line.

	Ch. 1	*Ch. 4*	*Ch. 8*		
80				80	*Extremely*
70				70	
60				60	*Highly*
50				50	
40				40	*Moderately*
30				30	
20				20	*Barely*
10				10	
0				0	
-10				-10	
-20				-20	*Ideally*
-30				-30	
-40				-40	*Mildly*
-50				-50	
-60				-60	*Overly*
-70				-70	*Excessively*
-80				-80	

Use a dot (•) for the (+) scores and an (x) for the (-) scores.
Now connect the dots with one line and connect the x's with another.

Compare these lines. Have your scores changed since Chapters One and Four? Have they gone down? Gone up? Stayed the same?

Now answer these questions:
*Before Chapter One, what was your positive energy level? _____
What is it now? _____*

*Before Chapter One, what was your negative energy level? _____
What is it now? _____*

After Chapters One, Two and Three, what was your positive energy level as you started Chapter Four? _____

After Chapters One, Two and Three, what was your negative energy level as you started Chapter Four? _____

*After Chapter Four, Five, Six and Seven, what was your positive energy level as you started Chapter Eight? _____
What would you like it to be? _____*

*After Chapters Four, Five, Six and Seven, what was your negative energy level as you started Chapter Eight? _____
What would you like it to be? _____*

If you want to reinforce positive attitudes and behaviors for physical and mental health, it's important to emphasize positive statements by learning to overcome negative thoughts. The graph on page 8-7 shows you how everyday life can affect your energy level. Use it as a baseline as you continue through your various routines.

When you are successful at incorporating or eliminating these statements in or out of your thoughts and actions, you will be able to determine how you influence daily events.

Incorporate these statements into your daily thoughts and actions.
Positive Cognitive Component Statements

> I show good judgment when I experience trials in my life.

> I think of the pressure to meet deadlines as a challenge.

> I believe that if I persist I will overcome any obstacles.

> I avoid feeling out of control by assessing my wants and working to achieve them.

> I have the self-confidence to remain faithful to my values.

> I can stay on task to achieve a goal.

> I make sound decisions that keep me happy and relaxed in my life.

> I am able to achieve the goals I set for myself.

> I use incentives to keep me focused on my objectives.

> I make careful choices when I want to change any of my behaviors.

> I know the direction I want to go in my life and I have the motivation and support to get there.

Eliminate these statements from your daily thoughts and actions.
Negative Cognitive Component Statements

> I act in a way which is contrary to my common sense or my wishes.

> I feel uncertain about my daily life. I have no direction and can't seem to find one.

Incorporate these statements into how you feel and act.
Positive Emotional Component Statements

I have plenty of energy and I look forward to each day.

I feel confident that I can meet any challenge and can get what I want.

I feel excited, motivated and sure about my life.

When I want to reach a goal, I have the support I need.

I feel happy with the choices I have made in my life so far.

I know the directions I want to go in my life, and I have the motivation and support to get there.

Eliminate these statements from how you feel and act.
Negative Emotional Component Statements

I feel confused and/or hopeless.

Because I feel uneasy around others, I avoid socializing.

I have fears which make me hesitate to act upon my desires.

Other people can make me feel rushed, angry, stressed or worried.

There are periods where I lack the courage to act effectively.

I feel restless and edgy.

I feel upset when others don't acknowledge my daily efforts.

I have strong fears of situations I am powerless to control or avoid.

I feel uncertain about my daily life. I have no direction and can't seem to find one.

I have brief periods of excessive agitation.

When I feel frustrated with my daily life, I don't want to see other people. I would rather stay home to avoid any contact.

I feel depressed and down.

I find myself overeating when I feel stressed, depressed or lonely.

I feel unfocused and unmotivated. When I feel like this, I move too slowly to accomplish what I need to accomplish.

It's difficult for me to get pleasure out of life.

I have considered harming myself or committing suicide.

I feel like a failure at the tasks I set for myself.

Incorporate these statements into how you act.
Positive *Behavioral Component Statements*

I have plenty of energy and I look forward to each day.

I think of the pressure to meet deadlines as a challenge.

I avoid feeling out of control by assessing my wants and working to achieve them.

I stay rested and alert so I can achieve my objectives.

I use exercise to relieve the stress of depression.

When I feel overburdened or fatigued, I use a brief period of relaxation to rejuvenate myself.

I maintain a healthy daily nutritional intake.

I take vacations.

I enjoy interacting with others.

I am able to achieve the goals I set for myself.

I use incentives to keep me focused on my objectives.

I make careful choices when I want to change any of my behaviors.

I stay motivated when I have set goals for myself.

Eliminate these statements from your action.

Negative Behavioral Component Statements

I feel tired for no apparent reason.

I have difficulty falling asleep or sleeping through the night.

I have problems with my digestive system: either constipation or diarrhea.

I have difficulty maintaining my life the way it used to be.

When I feel frustrated with my daily life, I don't want to see other people. I would rather stay home to avoid any contact.

I find myself overeating when I feel stressed, depressed or lonely.

My sex drive has decreased or is less than I would like.

I feel unfocused and unmotivated. When I feel like this, I move too slowly to accomplish what I need to accomplish.

I use alcohol or drugs as a means of relaxation.

I wish I had taken a different direction earlier in my life.

I don't have enough time for my family or friends.

I have verbal disagreements with others.

When you can maintain your effort to incorporate the positive components and eliminate the negative components you increase your ability to move into physical and mental balance.

WORKOUT: CARDIOMUSCULAR INTENSITY

Cardiomuscular intensity is designed to affect deep muscle fibers.

Do you feel: ready and willing, motivated, excited, confident, resigned and clear-minded before you start your workout?

Do you feel: discouraged, dreading, pressed for time, anxious, not sure or don't want to think about it before you start your workout?

If you don't feel like the descriptions above, what combination of feelings do you have before you start your workout?

WALK/JOG   OR   BIKE

Time _____ *HR* _____		*Time* _____ *HR* _____	
*Start*_____		*Start*_____	
@ 6 min	_____	@ 6 min	_____
@12 min	_____	@ 12 min	_____
@18 min	_____	@ 18 min	_____
@20 min	_____	@ 20 min	_____
*Stop*_____		*Stop* _____	

Lower Body Routine
1. Leg squats - 2 sets of 20 reps with no weight
Rest for 30 seconds after the first and 60 second after the second set

2. Walking Lunges - 2 sets of 20 reps each leg with no weight
Rest for 60 seconds after the first and second set

3. *Adductor (inner thighs) - 2 sets of 20 reps*
Small builds use 5 – 20 lbs if using leg pulley or ankle weights or use 20 – 50 lbs if using an adductor machine
Large builds use 10 – 20 lbs if using leg pulley or ankle weights or use 40 – 80 lbs if using an adductor machine
Rest for 30 seconds after the first second set

*5. Standing Alternating Leg Curls or Lying Leg Curls -
 2 sets of 20 reps*
Smaller builds use 10 - 20 lbs of ankle weights or 20 - 40 lbs
Larger builds use 20 - 30 lbs of ankle weights or 40 - 70 lbs
Rest for 30 seconds after the first and second set

6. Seated Leg Extension - 2 sets of 20 reps
Smaller builds use 20 lbs of ankle weights or on a machine
use 20- 40 lbs
Larger builds use 30 lbs of ankle weights or on a machine
use 40 - 70 lbs
Rest for 30 seconds after the first and second set and check
your heart rate after the second set: _____

7. Standing One Leg Calf Raises - 2 sets of 20 reps, with no weights

8. Flat Back Leg Raises - 1 set of 100 reps with no weights

*9. Flat Back Crunch Ups - 1 set of 100 reps with no weight,
Don't rest between reps*

*10. Side Crunch Ups - 1 sets of 75 reps with no weight,
Don't rest between reps*

*11. Flat Stomach Back Raises - 1 set of 100 reps with no weight
Don't rest between reps*

*Complete today's session by doing your stretching exercise
for 30 seconds each.*

*Did you feel you could have gone on forever, felt good after it was
over, like how you're feeling, energetic, active, powerful.*

Did you feel invigorated during your workout?

*Did you feel you needed more energy, had too many negative
thoughts, needed a partner or just wasn't interested during your
workout?*

Trainer's Comments & Suggestions:

A DAY FOR MASSAGE

Remember that a massage is an important step in your effort to achieve balance, because it is part of the self-awareness you will need to maintain a healthy body. Exercise, making informed decisions about your eating and learning to recognize the difference between a tense body and a relaxed one are all essential. Without them, any changes you make will be temporary. Taking the time to have a massage is an investment in your ongoing well-being.

Make sure you put this book by your bed tonight because there will be questions to answer before getting up. Have you made progress with your time schedule? How are your actual times comparing with your goal times?

ANKLE/ARM BLOOD PRESSURE RATE

The ankle to arm BP ratio is easily done by checking the blood pressure in the leg (over the posterior tibial artery) and comparing it to the blood pressure in the arm. Simply take the systolic pressure obtained in the arm and in the leg. Divide the leg systolic BP by the arm systolic BP. A low value (below 0.9) means a three times greater overall risk of death in the next 4 years without treatment, including 4 times greater risk of death from heart disease and 3 times greater risk from cancer. Have your doctor check this ratio for you. These studies were done in elderly people, so we're not yet certain if they can be extended to everyone. However, if you're younger and this ratio is low, it at least warrants further investigation by your doctor.

DAY 51   TODAY'S DATE:

Answer these questions before you get out of bed in the morning:
How did you feel when you woke up?

Did you get enough sleep?   Yes   No   If no, why not?

How did your dreams make you feel about yourself?

If a dream or event affected you negatively, what do you need to work on today to help you think more positively about yourself?

Answer these questions before you leave home:
How do you feel as you leave for school or work?

Do you feel motivated and clear about what you want to accomplish today? If not, what can you do to change this?

WORKOUT: CARDIOMUSCULAR INTENSITY
Upper Body Routine

R O W		W A L K / J O G OR B I K E	
Time _____ *HR* _____		*Time* _____ *HR* _____	
*Start*_____		*Start*_____	
@ 6 min	_____	@ 6 min	_____
@12 min	_____	@ 12 min	_____
@18 min	_____	@ 18 min	_____
@20 min	_____	@ 20 min	_____
*Stop*_____		*Stop* _____	

1. Seated Lat Rows 2 sets of 20 reps
Smaller builds use 20 to 60 lbs
Larger builds use 50 to 100 lbs
Rest for 30 seconds after the first and second set

2. Push-ups or Chest Press- 2 sets of 20 reps
Smaller builds use 20 to 40 lbs
Larger builds use 40 to 100 lbs
Rest for 30 seconds after the first set and second set

3. Lat Pull Downs - 2 sets of 20 reps
Smaller builds use 20 to 40 lbs
Larger builds use 50 to 110 lbs
Rest for 30 seconds after the first and second set

4. Flat Bench Chest Flies - 2 sets of 20 reps
Smaller builds use 3 to 10 lbs
Larger builds use 10 to 60 lbs
Rest for 30 seconds after the first and second set

5. Side Lateral Raises - 2 sets of 20 reps, with dumbbells
Smaller builds use 3 to 10 lbs
Larger builds use 15 to 25 lbs
Rest for 30 seconds after the first and second set

6. Triceps Push Downs - 2 sets of 20 reps
Smaller builds use 10 to 40 lbs
Larger builds use 30 to 60 lbs
Rest for 30 seconds after the second set

7. One Arm Biceps Curls - 2 sets of 20 reps, using dumbbells
Smaller builds use 5 to 15 lbs
Larger builds use 20 to 40 lbs
Rest for 30 seconds after the and second set

8. Forearm Curls / 2 sets of 20 reps
Smaller builds use 10 - 20 lbs
Larger builds use 20 - 40 lbs
Rest for 30 seconds after the first set

9. Flat Back Leg Raises–1 set of 100 reps

10. Flat Back Crunch Ups–1 set of 100 reps

11. Side Crunches–1 set of 100 reps

12. Flat Stomach Back Ups–1 set of 100 reps
Hold stretches for 30 seconds each.

Trainer's Comments & Suggestions:

EXAMINING THE INFLUENCES IN YOUR DAILY LIFE

Before you go to sleep tonight, think back over your day. What actions did you take to rid yourself of the negative influences? What did you experience today that made you feel enthusiastic and excited.

ANABOLIC STEROIDS

Anabolic steroids are a definite no. A program for strengthening, toning, fitness, body building or any other type of workout must not involve the use of anabolic steroids. One must be careful not to take "Amino Acids" or "Energizers" that might have some degree of anabolic steroids in them.

Anabolic steroids in men can cause decreased sperm count, testicular atrophy (decrease in size), hypertension, breast enlargement, acne, balding, low HDL cholesterol, high LDL cholesterol and cancer of the liver. In women, they can cause masculinization, menstrual irregularities, clitoral enlargement, decreased breast size, acne, deepened voice, and increased growth of facial hair and body hair. Many psychological side effects can also occur in both men and women. These include hyperactivity, irritability, aggressiveness and euphoria. Withdrawal from steroids causes depression, guilt, difficulty concentrating, excessive sleep and other psychiatric symptoms. Steroids are addictive. Many people who try to stop are drawn back to them because of the withdrawal symptoms.

DAY 52   TODAY'S DATE:
STAYING AWARE OF YOUR GOALS AND PERSEVERING

Remember, when you find yourself reacting to a situation in a way you don't like, choose to notice and learn. Now that you have reached this point in the book, look back.

What have you learned about yourself?

How have your thoughts and feelings affected you while you were going through Your Personal Trainer?

How do they affect you now?

What changes have you made?

KEEPING PERSPECTIVE IN YOUR LIFE

Both perceptions and attitudes contribute to your daily functioning. How you think and the way you feel about yourself will have a positive or negative effect on everything you do.

At the beginning of this book, we talked about the difference between thinking you should do something and knowing you are doing it. Understanding and acting on this concept allows you to have success in reaching any goal you set for yourself. In the first section of this book there is a list of possible wants. These include ways you may wish you could be or ways you think you should be.

Following is the same list, reworded as statements of fact.

Notice how these statements affect you:

I am in charge of my life.

How I appear and how I feel are the same.

As I get older, I am staying healthy and energetic.

I accept myself.

I am proud of my appearance.

I am proud of my accomplishments.

I enjoy my life and I am happy with what I have.

I am self-motivated and I don't compare myself with others.

I am learning to be relaxed.

I am becoming fit enough to take hikes and not be exhausted.

I have energy and stamina.

I am moving gracefully.

I am developing muscle tone and vitality.

My own character and style are showing through.

I have boldness and conviction in my walk.

I have dreams and goals.

I am facing my life with optimism, not depression.

I have good friends.

I have serenity and peace.

I am learning to know myself.

I am feeling and looking confident.

I am healthier and more fit.

I look forward to my workouts.

I am losing inches and toning my body.

I am losing weight and my body is looking the way I want it to look.

I am making sure I have the time to adjust to major changes in my life, such as medical problems, my job, money problems, family problems, etc.

Are there any other ways you have changed or any other observations you can make about your life now? Write them in the spaces.

I am _____

I am _____

I am _____

I am _____

I am _____

I am _____

I have _____

Look back over the two lists and write down the ten most important items for you. Read these every day. Some of these may not be entirely true yet, but if you work on them consciously, you will find your attitudes will change. Combine this list with the daily thought of:

> *In some small way, I will do something to improve myself each day of my life.*

DAY 53   TODAY'S DATE:
WORKOUT: CARDIOMUSCULAR INTENSITY

Upper Body Routine
How do you feel before starting your workout?

☐ Motivated   ☐ Discouraged   ☐ Clear-minded

☐ Excited   ☐ Dreading   ☐ Ready and willing

☐ Pressed for time   ☐ Resigned   ☐ Confident

☐ Anxious   ☐ Not sure   ☐ Don't want to
                                                 think about it

Do you know why you're doing this.   *Yes   No   Explain:*

How do these answers compare to your previous ones?
Is there a difference?   *Why?*

R O W		**W A L K / J O G O R B I K E**	
Time _____ *HR* _____		*Time* _____ *HR* _____	
*Start*_____		*Start*_____	
@ 6 min	____	@ 6 min	____
@12 min	____	@ 12 min	____
@18 min	____	@ 18 min	____
@20 min	____	@ 20 min	____
*Stop*_____		*Stop* _____	

Are you drinking enough water?

Follow upper body routine for Day 51. (pages, 16 -18)
Perform Stretches for 30 second each.

How did you feel during your workout?

☐ I needed more energy   ☐ I had too many negative thoughts

☐ I could have gone on forever ☐ I felt good after it was over

☐ I like how I'm feeling   ☐ I need a partner

☐ I just wasn't interested today ☐ I felt powerful

☐ What an invigorating feeling ☐ It's good to have my body active

Were you able to keep yourself motivated? If so, how? If not, why not?

How do you feel now that your workout is finished?

☐ Glad it's over   ☐ A feeling of accomplishment

☐ Can't wait until next time   ☐ Dreading next time

☐ I wish I'd started this long ago ☐ I understand its importance

☐ I feel rejuvenated   ☐ I feel successful

☐ Joyful   ☐ I didn't like doing this

I think and feel I am on my way to becoming more fit.
    Yes   *No*   *Explain:*

Trainer's Comments & Suggestions:

Remember the fourteen items that were listed as obstacles you may encounter when you try to start or maintain a physical fitness routine. You were to rank them from most (1) to least (14 or higher) likely to prevent you from reaching your goal(s). How do you rank them now?

____Time	____Family responsibilities
____Cost	____Pain/discomfort
____Embarrassment	____Knowing what to do
____Fatigue	____Inconvenience
____Weather	____Other people
____Transportation	____Lack of proper facilities
____Work	____Lack of family support

Notice the top three.
Can you think of solutions for these?
Write your ideas here:

A TIME FOR SILENCE

Today you'll be combining physical exercise with your meditation routine. Your goal for this time is to try to free your mind of any distracting thoughts. Give yourself this opportunity to step away from your life and gain perspective on how you are feeling and what affects those feelings. Now follow the directions for meditation I or II.

DAY 54   TODAY'S DATE:
WORKOUT ROUTINE: CARDIOMUSCULAR INTENSITY
Lower Body Routine

WALK/JOG	OR	BIKE
Time _____ *HR* _____		*Time* _____*HR* _____
*Start*_____		*Start*_____
@ 6 min _____		@ 6 min _____
@12 min _____		@ 12 min _____
@18 min _____		@ 18 min _____
@20 min _____		@ 20 min _____
*Stop*_____		*Stop* _____

Are you drinking enough water?

Follow Lower body routine for Day 50 (pages, 13 -14)
Perform stretches for 30 second each.

Trainer's Comments & Suggestions:

VITAMIN C & VITAMIN E

Vitamin C is an effective antioxidant which may help prevent various cancers in the body. It may also play some role in prevention of coronary disease. Though controversial, regular vitamin C intake may reduce the severity and duration of the common cold. We generally recommend the intake of 500-1000mg. per day of vitamin C either through nutritional intake or supplementation.

Vitamin E has long been treated as a very beneficial vitamin. It has antioxidants effects that may reduce the risk of some cancers and may also decrease the risk of coronary artery disease. Should you use supplements? Many people are now supplementing with 400 IU per day. Vitamin E and C remain controversial but, increasingly, evidence indicates they are highly beneficial. It may be best to get them from your food. However, if you find it difficult to consistently get them in your normal nutritional intake, a 500 mg. tablet and a 400 IU vitamin E are recommended.

DAY 55   TODAY'S DATE:
STAYING AWARE OF YOUR GOALS AND PERSEVERING

Answer these questions before you get out of bed in the morning:
How did you feel when you woke up?

Did you get enough sleep?   Yes   No   If no, why not?

How did your dreams make you feel about yourself?

If a dream or event affected you negatively, what do you need to work on today to help you think more positively about yourself?

Answer these questions before you leave home:
How do you feel as you leave for school or work?

Do you feel motivated and clear about what you want to accomplish today?   If not, what can you do to change this?

Answer these questions when you return home:
How did you feel during your day?

Did you plan all your activities for the day? Yes   or   No

Were you able to stay with these plans?   Yes   or   No
If no, what happened?

What could you do next time to prevent this from happening?

Answer these questions at the end of your day:
How do you feel as the day is ending?

Did you accomplish what you wanted to accomplish? Explain.

If you weren't able to reach your goals, what steps could you take to help yourself come closer tomorrow?

Remember, just as you have created negative habits, you are now creating positive ones. You are learning to replace old responses with positive ones. You also know that if you find yourself reacting to a situation in a way you don't like, you can choose to notice and learn.

MEDITATION: A TIME FOR SILENCE

Today is a day off from physical exercise. Instead, you will take the time to relax. As you go through the day, remember to notice how your energy is being affected by events and people. As you meditate, and take time for silence free your mind of any concerns or anxieties. Increase your meditation to 30 minutes. Choose meditation routine I or II.

Take time out today for a massage. An experienced masseur or masseuse can keep you informed about body and how your exercise and daily life are affecting it. Take the time to relax and enjoy the feeling of relaxation.

DAY 56   TODAY'S DATE:
SELF REFLECTION

As you've worked your way through *Your Personal Trainer*, you've examined the ways in your behavior, perception and your attitude can be affected by daily life. You may have noticed that there are cycles to your feelings and therefore cycles in your experiences. For example, if someone makes a comment to you and your feelings are hurt, you react. You may get angry. You may withdraw or you may ask questions. Whatever you do, you will be affected. The result of this may be that you eat more or less, exercise more or less, interact more or less. However you react, the awareness of this reaction will help you to prevent the repetition of behaviors that could be harmful to you.

Learning how you are is the first step to learning who you are. *Your Personal Trainer* has made you aware of the many solutions you can use to face daily influences. Before you started this routine, you decided you wanted to change. You may have been unhappy with your weight, your fitness level, your looks or just your general feelings about yourself. Although it may have been difficult during the last 56 days, you have persevered. Congratulations.

WHAT HAVE YOU LEARNED?

During the last fifty-five days, you have learned to pay attention to how you're feeling, what your thoughts are, and how you use your time. You have increased your cardiovascular endurance and toned your body. You have learned various facts about health, nutrition and your emotional state. You have examined how you feel and think before, during and after you exercise. You have learned how it feels to take care of yourself, both physically and emotionally. We hope you will want to continue to do this.

Your Personal Trainer has taught you how to balance and control physical and mental efforts by focusing and concentrating on making your life better. Now that you have gone through the book, we hope you will take what you have learned about yourself and apply it as a lifelong effort. As you have already discovered, changing long held beliefs and attitudes about yourself can be difficult.

Let's take a look at what you have done in order to understand how you can maintain your active approach towards feeling and thinking fit.

During Chapters One and Two you concentrated on establishing and strengthening your foundation by beginning to workout aerobically, walking/ jogging or biking, independently or combining them into one workout. You finished with cardiomuscular flexibility stretches to elongate your muscles and prevent shortening of the ligaments and tendons.

Chapter Three had you concentrating on challenging yourself by combining aerobic exercise (walking/jogging or biking) with one set of strengthening exercises, performing 12 repetitions for each exercise. You stretched each muscle used. These exercises were done at your home or in a club or gym. You finished your workout by concentrating on working your abdominal area (lower, upper, sides and back) with sets of 25.

During Chapter Four you concentrated on taking control of your life by continuing to combine aerobic exercise with strengthening exercises. These exercises were also done at home or in a club or gym. You finished your workout by working your abdominal area as you did in Chapters One, Two and Three.

When you made it to Chapter Five, you set realistic goals by continuing to combine aerobic exercise with two sets of strengthening exercises. These exercises were also done at home or in a club or gym. You finished your workout by again working your abdominal area as you did in Chapters One, Two, Three and Four.

In Chapter Six, you concentrated on making permanent changes by continuing to combine aerobic exercise with strengthening exercises. You started your strengthening workout by working your abdominal area lower, upper, sides and back with sets of 50 repetitions for each exercise. You finished your overall workout with stretches for each muscle you'd exercised. These exercises were also done at your home or in a club or gym.

While Chapter Six tested your perseverance, Chapters Seven and Eight tested your intensity. In these you concentrated on staying on track and staying healthy and fit as a way of life by continuing to combine aerobic exercise with two sets of strengthening exercises. You finished these by working your abdominal area (lower, upper, sides and back) with a set of 100 repetitions for each exercise. You finished your overall workout with stretches for each muscle you'd exercised. These exercises were also done at your home or in a gym or club.

> *Look again at your daily schedule, have you been planning your time wisely? How close are your actual times to your goal times?*

CHAPTER NINE

STRETCHES / EXERCISES
HOME WORKOUT
GYM/CLUB WORKOUT

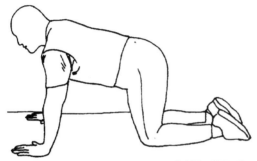

CAT STRETCH

Get on your hands and knees. Begin by arching your back. Hold for the assigned time. Make sure you are feeling the stretch in your lower back. Half way through your count, start to lean back. Complete your stretch by sitting on your buttocks.

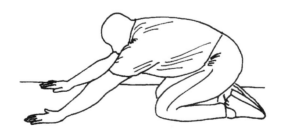

KNEELING QUADRICEPS STRETCH

Sit upright on your knees with your back straight. Place both hands on the floor behind you, fingers facing outward. Lean back and raise your buttocks, feeling the stretch in the front of your thighs. Hold for the assigned time.

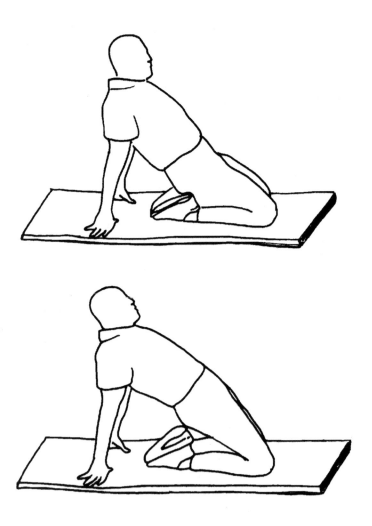

QUADRICEPS/HIP FLEXOR-HAMSTRING STRETCH

Do this stretch after you finished your kneeling quadriceps stretch. You will finish with both hands and knees on the floor. Start this stretch by putting one leg forward. Then place both arms on the inside of your body, with your hands close to your front foot. Lean forward making sure you feel the stretch in your quads and hip flexor. Hold the stretch for the assigned time.

Hamstrings stretch—Lean backward and put both hands on each side of the leg. Make sure you lean back enough so your toes are pointing to the ceiling. Feel the stretch in the back of your leg. Hold the stretch for the assigned time. Repeat this with the other leg.

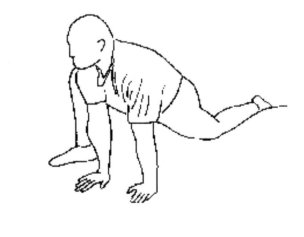

OBLIQUE/ADDUCTOR/ HAMSTRINGS/ STRETCH

Sit on your buttocks, extend one leg out straight and bring the opposite foot into the adductor area (inside thigh) of the straight leg. Place one hand on the inner part of the knee that is bent, then grasp the foot of the stretched out leg. Press down on the inner part of the knee and pull on the foot of the stretched out leg. Hold the stretch for the assigned time.

Repeat with the other leg.

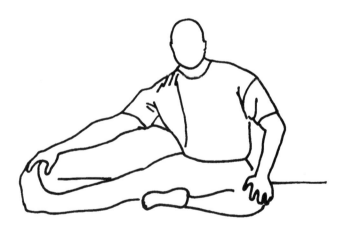

STRAIGHT LEG STRETCH (SIT AND REACH)

Sit on your buttocks and extend both legs out straight. Grasp both of your feet. Make sure you feel the stretch in your legs and not in your lower back. Hold the stretch for the assigned time.

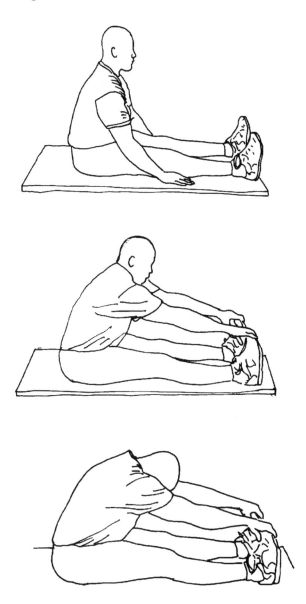

ADDUCTOR STRETCH

Sit on your buttocks and bring both feet as close to the buttocks as possible. Grasp both ankles and place both elbows on the inner side of the knees. Press down on the knees with the elbows.

Hold the stretch for the assigned time.

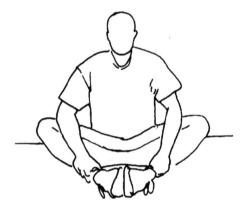

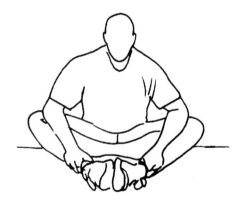

GLUTEUS MAXIMUS STRETCH

Sit on your buttocks and cross one leg over to the outside of the opposite leg. Keeping it aligned with the knee of the straight leg. Place both hands on the knee that is near the chest. Pull and press the knee with both hands.

Hold the stretch for the assigned time.

Follow the same directions for the other leg.

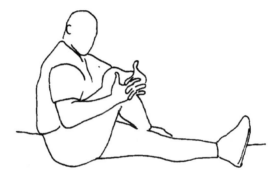

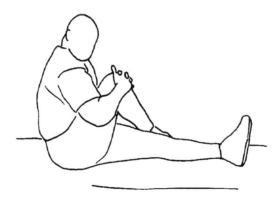

OBLIQUE STRETCH

Start this stretch as if you are doing the gluteus stretch. However, you will take both arms and twist to the opposite position of your legs. Place both hands on the floor and gently twist your body so you will feel the stretch in your oblique. Make sure you keep your upper body in a straight line. Hold the stretch for the assigned time. Follow the same directions for the other leg.

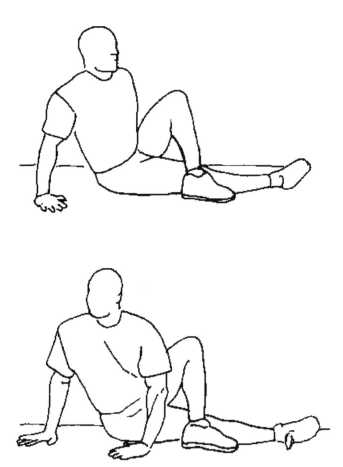

LOWER BACK STRETCH

Lie flat on the floor. Extend one arm over your head. Bring one leg over the other leg and take hold of the knee with your hand. You should feel the stretch in your lower back and in your pectoral muscles. You can adjust the leg with the knee up or down to receive the full range of the stretch. Move the arm to the right or left of your head in order to receive the full range of this stretch. Hold the stretch for the assigned time. Follow the same instructions for the other leg.

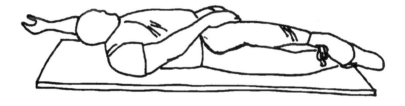

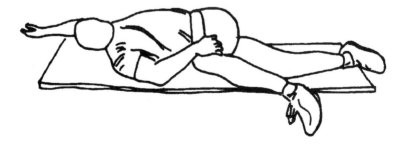

LATISSIMUS DORSI STRETCH

Standing in front of a vertical bar, grab the bar with both hands. Bend your knees as if you are doing a squat. Lean back while holding the bar and feel the stretch in your lats. Hold the stretch for the assigned time. Slowly stand up and make sure your arms are parallel to the floor. Pull back and feel the stretch in the upper part of your back. Hold the stretch for the assigned time.

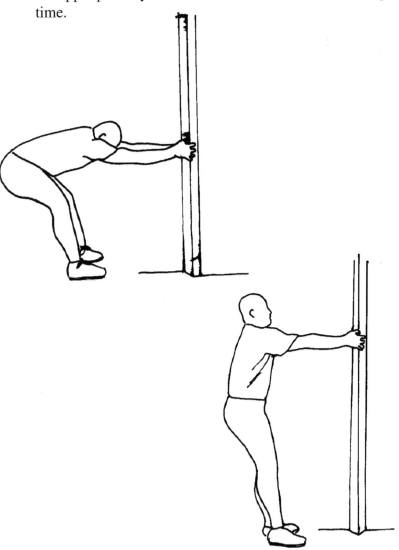

PECTORALS/BICEPS STRETCH

Standing in an oblique position with a vertical bar behind your, place the palm of your hand on the bar, make sure your arm is extended. Do not grab the bar tightly. Press outward from the bar and feel the stretch in the chest muscle. Hold the stretch for the assigned time. Follow the same instruction for the other side.

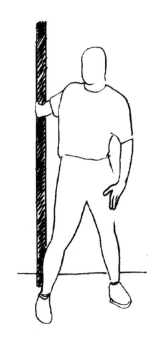

TRICEPS STRETCH

Standing straight – place one arm over your head. Let your arm bend at the elbow and place your hand in the small of your back. Take the other hand and grab the elbow and pull the arm towards your head. Hold the stretch for the assigned time. Follow the same instruction for the other side.

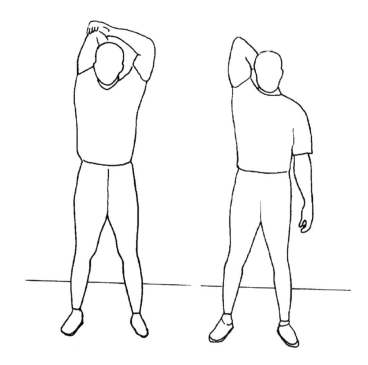

WORKOUT: LOWER BODY ROUTINE

STANDING ALTERNATING LEG CURLS

What to do:

Strap on the ankle weights. Stand in front of a high back chair. Place your hands on the back of the chair. Raise your leg while bending at the knee. In order to concentrate and isolate the hamstring, make sure you're pointing your foot outward. After you have completed one leg, do the same movement with the other leg. It is important with this exercise that you focus on exhaling as you lift your leg and inhaling as you lower your leg. Take slow and controlled breaths. If you do not have a leg curl machine at home, do these exercises.

What to expect:

As you perform reps 1 through 5, concentrate on proper body and leg alignment. Between reps 5 and 8 you will become aware of your hamstring muscles. This awareness will begin to be more pronounced between reps 9 and 12 and your hamstring muscles will begin to feel tight.

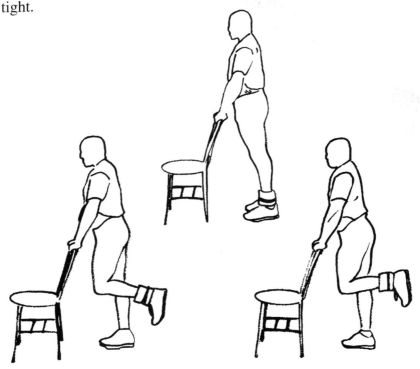

LYING LEG CURLS

What to do:
This is an excellent exercise for slowly warming up your leg muscles. Stand in front of the leg curl machine, straddling the leg rollers. Lie down on your stomach and insert your feet beneath the rollers. Place your hands on the protruding bar handles on both sides of the bench. This will help keep you in a tight position. Raise your legs while bending at the knee. Take slow and controlled breaths. Focus on *exhaling* as you lift your legs and *inhaling* as you carefully lower them. By pointing your feet outward this exercise will have an isolated and concentrated effect on your hamstrings. This may be a little difficult for a beginner. If so, start by pointing your feet down.

What to expect:
As you perform reps 1 through 5, concentrate on proper body and leg alignment. Between reps 5 and 8 you will become aware of your hamstring muscles. Between reps 9 and 12 you may start to feel a burning sensation in your hamstring muscles.

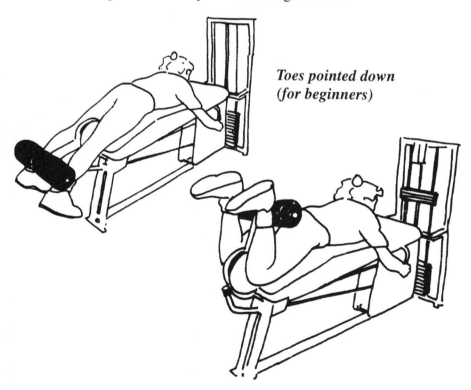

Toes pointed down (for beginners)

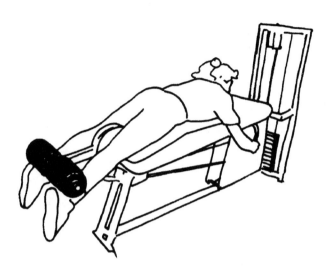

*toes pointed outward
(advanced)*

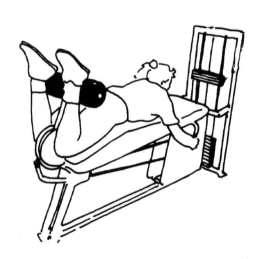

SEATED LEG EXTENSIONS (W/ANKLE WEIGHTS)

What to do:

Strap on your ankle weights. Sit erect in a chair
or on a bench. With one leg remaining on the
floor, lift the other leg up. As you raise the
leg, pay close attention to the sensation that
this movement creates. Don't lock your knee
at the top of the exercise. However, squeeze
your thigh once you get your leg just under
parallel to the floor. Again, *exhale* as you lift
your leg and *inhale* as you lower it. Be sure to
take slow and controlled breaths. If you have
had knee injuries or if you experience any discomfort using weights for this exercise, do the
leg movements without weights. If you do not
have a leg extension machine at home, do this
exercise.

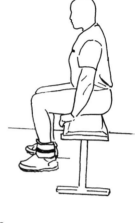

What to expect:

Between reps 1 and 8, check your body
alignment. Are your thighs straight? Are
your knees not leaning to either side?
Between reps 9 and 12 you will start to
feel a slight burning sensation in your
quadriceps. This is normal.

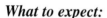

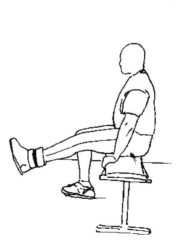

SEATED LEG EXTENSIONS (MACHINE)

What to do:

The seated leg extension is excellent for the front part of your legs although it can be a strain on your knees. If you experience pain in your knees, discontinue this exercise and consult your doctor. If you find it uncomfortable with the suggested weight, try lowering the weight. You will begin this exercise by sitting on the leg extension machine, make sure you have your lower back flush with the upper board. With both ankles under the rollers, lift both feet up. As you do this, pay lose attention to the sensation the movement creates. Don't lock your knees at the top of the exercise. However, you should squeeze your thighs once you get your legs just under parallel to the floor. *Exhale* as you lift your legs and *inhale* as you lower them. Make sure your breathing is slow and controlled.

What to expect:

Between reps 1 and 4, check your body alignment. Are your thighs parallel to one another? Between reps 5 and 8, you may start to feel burning in your quadriceps. This is normal. Between reps 9 and 12 your quadriceps may start to feel tighter.

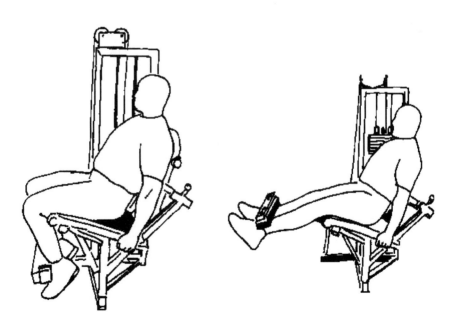

SQUATS

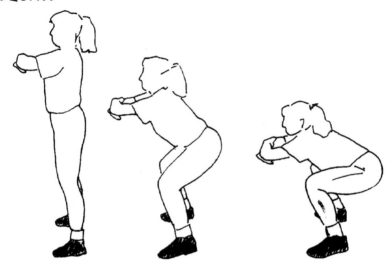

What to Do:

The squat is an excellent exercise to work the whole body. If you experience pain in your knees, discontinue this exercise and consult your doctor. You will be working your legs primarily, but there are also secondary muscles which are worked, including abdomen, back and chest. It's not important to use weights with this exercise in this program. Your main objective is to concentrate on your form. You will begin this exercise by positioning your feet about shoulder width apart. Fold your arms in front of your chest. Slowly begin to bend your knees, as if you are going to sit in a chair. Lower yourself down, keeping in mind that you want to keep your knees from going over your toes. Don't lock your knees at the top of the exercise or go past parallel to the floor. Make sure you squeeze your thighs as you straighten your legs. Exhale as you come up and inhale as you lower yourself to the floor. Make sure your breathing is slow and controlled.

What to expect:

Between reps 1 and 4, check your body alignment. Are you keeping your back slightly bent when you go down? Are your knees not leaning to either side? Are you keeping your knees from going over your toes in the down position. Between reps 5 and 8, you may start to feel burning in your quadriceps. This is normal. Between reps 9 and 12, your quadriceps may start to feel tighter. Between reps 13 and 15 you may begin to breath more heavily. Between the 15th and 20th repetitions, your quadriceps will feel very hot. This feeling is due to the amount of blood you are pumping into your legs. The exercise may feel difficult at this time, but persevere and you will receive the benefits of tight legs and buttocks.

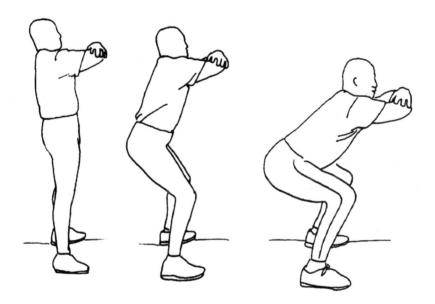

STATIONARY LUNGES
What to Do:
The stationary lunge is an excellent exercise to develop the quadriceps and buttocks. Because the movement can be extremely hard on the knees, make sure to you maintain your alignment. However, if you, experience pain in your knees, discontinue this exercise and consult your doctor. It's not important to use weights with this exercise in this program. Your main objective is to concentrate on your form. You will begin this exercise by positioning one of your legs in front of you. Put your hands on your hips, keeping your upper body straight. Lower yourself, keeping in mind your front knee shouldn't go over your toes. Your back leg should be bent so your knee goes down but stops before it touches the floor. Make sure you squeeze your front thigh as you ascend to the top of the movement. Don't lock your knees when you return to the up position. Alternate each leg. Exhale as you come up and inhale as you lower yourself to the floor. Make sure your breathing is slow
and controlled.

What to expect:
Between reps 1 and 4, check your body alignment. Are you keeping your back straight? Are your knees in a straight line? Are you keeping your knees from going over your toes in the down position. Between reps 5 and 8, you may start to feel burning in your quadriceps. This is normal. Between reps 9 and 12, your quadriceps may start to feel tighter. Between reps 13 and. 15, you may begin to breath more heavily. However, between the 15th and the 20th repetitions your quadriceps will feel very hot. This feeling is due to the amount of blood you are pumping into your legs. The exercise may feel difficult at this time, but persevere and you will receive the benefits of tight legs and buttocks.

ALTERNATING LUNGES

What to Do:

The alternating lunge is an excellent exercise to develop the quadriceps and buttocks. Because the movement can be extremely hard on the knees, make sure you maintain your alignment. However, if you experience pain in your knees, discontinue this exercise and consult your doctor. It's not important to use weights with this exercise in this program. Your main objective is to concentrate on your form. You will begin this exercise by standing straight. Put your hands on your hips, keeping your upper body straight. Step out with one leg and lower yourself, keeping in mind your front knee shouldn't go over your toes. Your back leg should be bent so your knee goes down but stops before it touches the floor. Make sure you squeeze your front thigh as you ascend to the top of the movement. Don't lock your knees when you return to the up position. Alternate each leg for the assigned number of reps. Exhale as you come up and inhale as you lower yourself to the floor. Make sure your breathing is slow and controlled.

What to expect:

You should expect basically the same as you would in doing the stationary lunges, except because of your movement back and forth, you will breathe much harder.

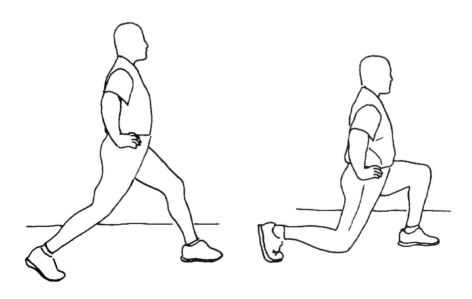

WALKING LUNGES

What to Do:

The walking lunge is an excellent exercise to develop the quadriceps, buttocks, and improve your cardiovascular endurance and intensity. Because the movement can be extremely hard on the knees, make sure you maintain your alignment. However, if you experience pain in your knees, discontinue this exercise and consult your doctor. It's not important to use weights with this exercise in this program. Your main objective is to concentrate on your form. You will begin this exercise by standing straight. Put your hands on your hips, keeping your upper body straight. Step out with one leg and lower yourself, keeping in mind your front knee shouldn't go over your toes. Your back leg should be bent so your knee goes down but stops before it touches the floor. Make sure you squeeze your front thigh as you straighten. Alternate walking each leg for the assigned number of reps. Exhale as you come up and inhale as you lower yourself to the floor. Make sure your breathing is slow and controlled.

What to expect:

You should expect basically the same as you would doing the stationary and alternating lunge, except because of your forward movement, you will breath much harder.

STANDING LEG ADDUCTOR (INNER THIGHS)

What to do:

To perform this exercise, you'll need the back of a chair or something else you can grasp at a comfortable height. Strap your ankle weights on and let both hands rest on the back of the chair. Keeping one leg stationary, use a sweeping motion to cross the other leg in front. Keep your moving leg slightly bent. After you finish, do the other leg the same way. Remember to exhale as you bring your leg across and inhale as the leg is returned to its original position. Your breathing should be slow and controlled, not labored. If you do not have a leg adductor machine at home, do this exercise.

What to expect:

During the first 8 reps you may not feel much response in your inner thigh. But between 9 and 12 reps, you should start to feel a tightening sensation within your inner thighs.

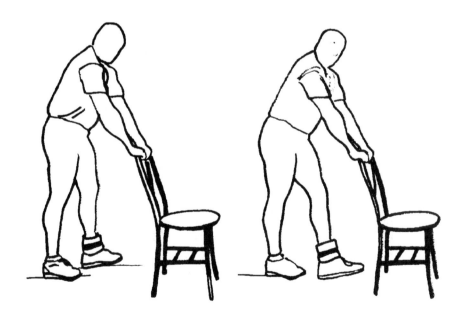

ADDUCTORS (INNER THIGHS)

What to do:

Stand in front of the leg apparatus, making sure you position the roller on the meaty part of your leg, just above the knee. Position your hands on the bars provided. Keeping your moving leg slightly bent, sweep it in front of the stationary leg. Remember to *exhale* as you sweep your leg in front and *inhale* as you return it to its original position. Perform the same movement with both legs.

What to expect:

During the first 8 reps you may not feel much response in your adductor. However, between reps 9 and 12, you may feel a tightening in your inner thighs.

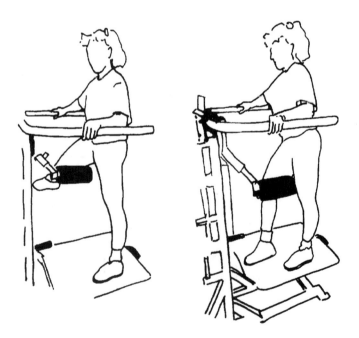

STANDING ONE LEG CALF RAISES

What to do:

To perform this exercise, you'll need the back of a chair or something else you can grasp at a comfortable height. Stand in front of the chair and gently place your hands on the top of it. Bend one of your legs at the knee and hold it there until you are done. Raise your other foot as high as you can, ending with standing on the ball of your feet. Lower your body, ending with your heel slightly off of the floor. Make sure that you aren't leaning to either side. Repeat this movement for the assigned number of repetitions. After you are done with one leg, repeat the same movement with the other leg. Remember to *exhale* as you lift yourself up on your ball of your feet and *inhale* as you lower yourself back to the original position. Your breathing should be slow and controlled, not labored.

What to expect:

During the first 10 reps, concentrate on your body alignment. As you perform these leg raises, you may feel a strong burning sensation in your calf muscle and up into your leg. This may be particularly true for the last 5 reps. But if possible, don't rest until you have completed all the reps.

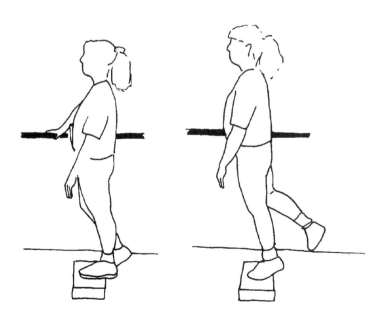

WORKOUT: MID SECTION EXERCISES

FLAT BACK LEG RAISES

What to do:
The flat stomach back raises will strengthen your lower abdomen. As with all of these exercises, it's important to concentrate on performing them correctly. Lie down on your back, raise your legs and bend them at the knees. Your feet should be on the floor. Position your arms by your body, then insert your hands, palms facing downward, under your buttocks. Start the exercise by raising your legs and feet off the floor, bending at the waist. Be sure that you concentrate on lifting with your abdomen. In order to isolate your lower abs its important that you lift you head and point it forward. You should only do this when you feel stronger and you have control of the exercise. *Exhale* as you bring your legs up and *inhale* as you lower them.

What to expect:
During the first 15 reps your neck may start to feel tight. If it starts to hurt, lay your head back down and take slow and controlled breaths. Try to relax your neck as you perform this exercise. Between reps 16 and 19 your back may start to burn and hurt. If so, stop and rest for 3-5 seconds. As you perform this exercise, you should be concentrating on feeling a burning sensation in your lower abdomen.

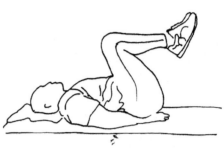

FLAT BACK CRUNCH UPS

What to do:
The flat stomach back raises will strengthen your lower abdomen. Lie down on your back, raise your legs and bend them at the knees. Your feet should be on the floor. Take a towel and wrap it around your neck. While holding the towel at both ends, cradle your head in the towel and raise your upper body. This is meant as a brace for your neck only, you shouldn't pull on it to help raise your head. Start the exercise by raising your upper torso off the floor, bending at the waist. Be sure that you concentrate on lifting with your abdomen. This is an excellent exercise for the upper stomach muscles. Exhale as your bring your upper body forward and inhale as you lower it to the floor.

What to expect:
During the first 15 reps your neck may feel a tightness in your neck muscles if you are pulling up with the towel. Try to concentrate on your breathing and on relaxing your neck in the cradle of the towel. Between reps 16 and 19 you may start to feel a burning sensation in your abs. You may also feel an increasing tightness in your neck. If so, try to relax your neck. If you find your neck continues to hurt, you may want to perform this exercise in blocks of 5's and 10's until you have completed the 25 reps.

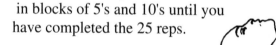

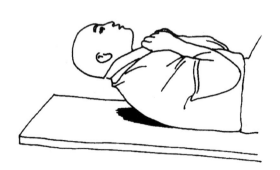

SIDE CRUNCH UPS

What to Do:

The side crunch ups will strengthen your oblique (side) muscles.
It's important to concentrate on performing this exercise correctly.
Start by lying on your side extending your arm in front of you, per-
pendicular to your body, palm facing up. Raise your upper arm and
curl your fingers around the back of your head. Slowly raise your
body off of the floor, as if you were doing a sideways sit-up. Remember to exhale as you bring your upper body forward and inhale
as you return to the starting position.

What to expect:

During the first 15 reps you should concentrate on your body
alignment. Between reps 16 and 19 you may start to feel a burning
feeling in your abs. If you can stay focused during reps 20 and 25,
you will have a more concentrated effect on your abdomen. However, if you become too uncomfortable, do the reps in sets of 5 or 10,
with a short rest of 15 seconds in between the sets. Rest for 30 seconds when you have completed this exercise.

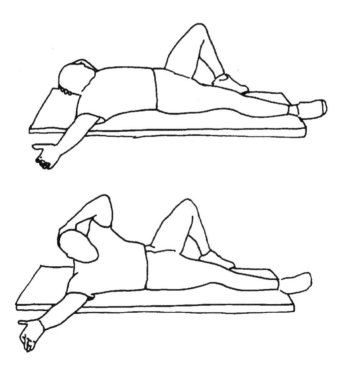

FLAT STOMACH BACK RAISES

What to do:
The flat stomach back raises will strengthen your lower back. As with all of these exercises, its important to concentrate on performing this exercise correctly. Lie face down, on your stomach, keeping your head in alignment with your back. Your arms should be positioned by your body with your palms facing upward. Start the exercise by raising your upper body off the floor, only bending at the waist. Be sure you don't lift your head before your shoulders. Exhale as you raise your body and inhale as you return to the starting position. Your breathing should be slow and controlled, no labored.

What to expect:
During the first 15 reps you may feel tightness in your lower back. Between reps 16 and 19 you may feel burning and pain in your lower back. Reps 20 and 25 may bring even more burning. If it's difficult to continue, take a 15 second rest and then finish the exercise.

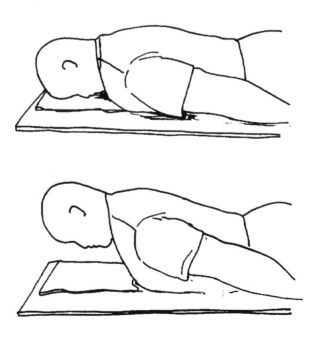

WORKOUT: UPPER BODY ROUTINE

BENT OVER ROWS

What to do:

If you experience pain in your lower back or have lower back problems, you may not want to do this exercise until you first consult with your doctor. Bend at the waist with your back parallel to the floor. Holding your dumbbell in one hand, place the opposite hand and knee on the bench. This will help support your back. Pull the weight to your chest and slowly extend your arm. Exhale as you pull the weight to your chest and inhale as you extend your arm. Be sure to control each movement. Maintain the correct positioning of your knee and hand on the bench. Keep the rest of your body as still as possible. If you do not have a lat row machine at home, do this exercise.

What to expect:

Between reps 9 and 12 your upper back may start to tighten. If possible, continue exercising without resting between reps.

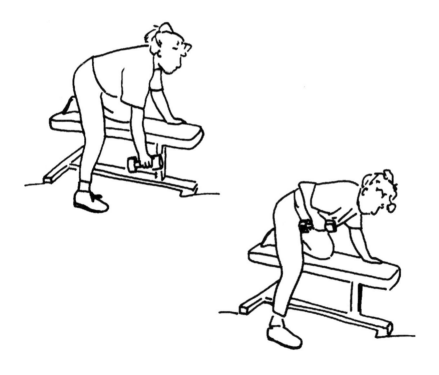

SEATED LAT ROWS

What to do:

Sit on the bench and take the bar in both hands. Lean forward and pull the weights off of the stack. Keep your arms extended but with your knees and elbows slightly bent. Squeezing your back muscles, slowly pull the weight to your chest. Then slowly lower the weights so that your arms are almost fully extended. Exhale as you pull the weight to your chest and inhale as you extend your arms again.

What to expect:

It's important to keep your back straight for this exercise. During reps 1 to 8 pay attention to your leg positions. Bend your knees so you keep the pressure off of your lower back. From reps 9 through 12, your back will begin to tighten.

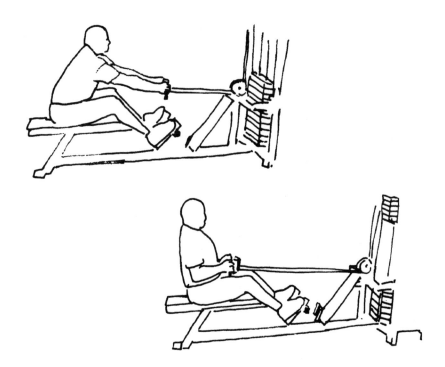

LAT PULL DOWNS

What to do:
With your back toward the apparatus, grasp the bar with both hands. Sit on the bench and extend your arms so your elbows are slightly bent. Squeezing your back muscles, pull the bar down so it just barely touches your shoulders. Slowly return the bar to the starting position. Make sure you keep your arms in line with your body. Keep movement from other parts of your body to a minimum. Keep your back straight and your feet in front of your body. Exhale as you pull the weights down and inhale as you let the weights return to their starting position.

What to expect:
During the first 8 reps your triceps and biceps may start to fatigue because you have just finished doing your chest exercises. However, try to maintain your effort because between reps 9 and 12 you may feel the effects of your effort with tightening of your back muscles.

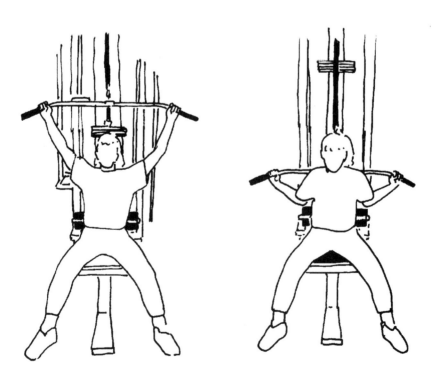

OVERHEAD LATERAL PULLS

What to do:

Lie face up on a flat bench. Grasp the dumbbell bar with both hands, extending your arms up above you. Keep your elbows slightly bent and position the bar so it's not directly above your face. Keeping your arms in the same position, slowly lower the bar behind your head. Your arms should be extended above your head, in line with your body. Slowly raise the weight back to its starting position. There should be minimal movement from the rest of your body. Adjust your hand position on the bar and the angle of your arms until you find a position that's not awkward and allows you to feel in control. In the starting position, be sure not to hold the weight over your face. Inhale as you lower the weight behind your head and exhale as you return to the starting position. If you do not have a lat pull down machine at home, do this exercise.

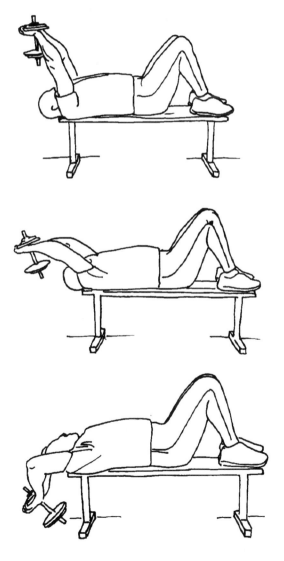

What to expect:

Between reps 1 and 8 concentrate on doing this exercise correctly. Between reps 9 and 12 your Lats, Triceps and Chest muscles may start to feel tight.

PUSH-UPS

What to do:
Initially you will be doing this exercise with your knees down.
Place your knees and hands on the floor, with your hands slightly
more than shoulder width apart. Keeping your body straight,
slowly lower your upper body until your face is just off of the
floor. Then slowly raise your body back to the starting position.
Inhale as you lower your face to the floor and exhale as you return
to the starting position. Keep your back flat, without sagging or
arching, and your body straight. This exercise can feel difficult
initially, but regular practice makes a difference.

What to expect:
You may feel a tightening and/or
burning sensation in your triceps
during the first 8 reps. Between reps
9 and 12 this feeling may intensify.

bent knee push-ups

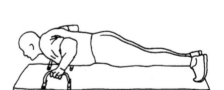

traditional push-ups

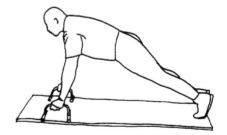

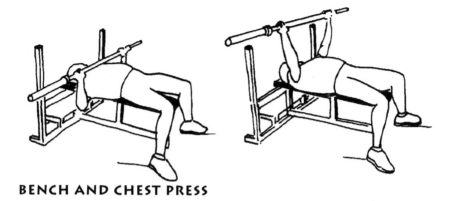

BENCH AND CHEST PRESS

What to do:
Take a seat on the bench. Lie back on the bench with your feet on the floor and grasp the bar with both hands. Make sure you align your hands on the bar so they are shoulder width apart. Lift the bar off of the rack. As you hold the bar over your head, slowly lower it to your chest. Don't let the bar touch your chest. Push the bar up, extending your arms while keeping your elbows slightly bent. Exhale as you extend your arms and inhale as you return your arms to the starting position. Your wrists should stay in line with your arms and hands. Keep your arms parallel with the floor. Your wrists should stay in line with your arms and your hands.

What to expect:
During the first 8 reps your triceps muscles may start to fatigue before your chest muscles do. Between 9 and 12 this feeling may intensify. Try to concentrate on the strength you are using and developing.

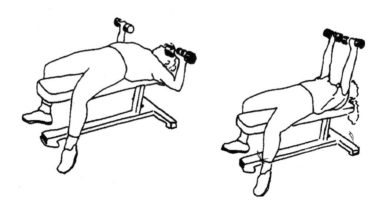

FLAT BENCH FLIES

What to do:
Lie flat on your back on a bench, with your feet on the floor and a dumbbell in each hand. Extend your arms above your chest, hands facing each other, keeping your elbows slightly bent. Maintaining the same elbow position, slowly lower your arms until your triceps are parallel to the floor. Then, slowly return your arms to the starting position. Remember to keep your elbows slightly bent by imagining you are hugging a barrel. Be conscious of using your chest muscles as you return the weights to the starting position. Inhale as you lower your arms and exhale as your return your arms to the starting position.

What to expect:
This exercise uses the same muscles as the push-ups, but at a different angle. Because of this, you may find these muscles more fatigued during the first 8 reps. Between reps 9 and 12, your chest may begin to feel tight.

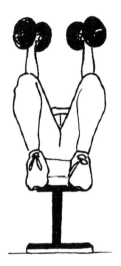

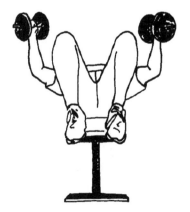

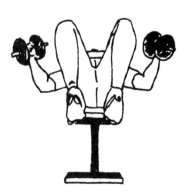

LATERAL DELTOID RAISES

What to do:
Sit on a flat bench, with your back straight. Holding one weight in each hand, let your arms hang down the side of your body, palms facing in. Slowly lift your arms until your arms are parallel with the floor. Keep your elbows slightly bent. Slowly return your arms to the starting position. This movement may feel awkward, so it's important to move slowly and carefully. Keep your back straight and your head facing forward. Exhale as you extend your arms and inhale as your return to the starting position.

What to expect:
During the first 8 reps you may feel a gradual tightening in your shoulders. Between reps 9 and 12 you may start to feel a burning sensation in your shoulders. If possible, finish your reps without resting in between reps.

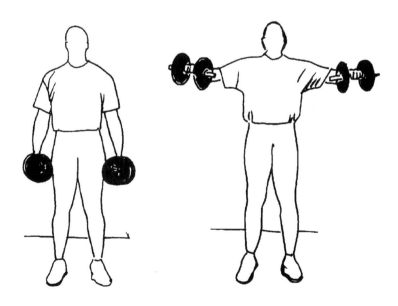

TRICEPS KICK BACKS

What to do:
Bend at the waist with your back parallel to the floor. For example, holding your dumbbell in your right hand, place your left hand and left knee on a bench for back support. When you switch the dumbbell to your left hand place your right hand and right knee on the bench for support. Pull the weight in, holding it so it's almost to your chest. Slowly, keeping it next to your side, extend your arm to the rear. Slowly bring your arm back to the starting position. Because of the angle of your arm, this exercise may feel awkward at first. Exhale as you extend your arm and inhale as your return it to the starting position. If you do not have a lat push down machine at home, do this exercise.

What to expect:
During the first 8 reps, watch your alignment and concentrate on keeping the rest of your body still. Between reps 9 and 12 you may feel a burning sensation in your triceps starting with your elbow and moving up to your shoulder. If you can, continue to exercise without resting.

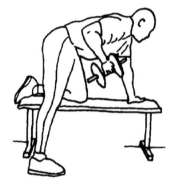 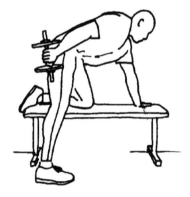

TRICEPS PUSH DOWN

What to do:
Grasp the bar and bend at the waist with your back slightly bent.
Holding your bar in front of your chest with both hands in your
right hand press down. It's important you keep your elbows locked
in at your side. Make sure your wrist is locked in a straight position
in line with your arm. Slowly bring your arms back to the starting
position. Exhale as you press down and inhale as you return to the
starting position. Because of the angle of your arm, this exercise
may feel awkward at first.

What to expect:
During the first 8 reps, watch your alignment and concentrate on
keeping the rest of your body still. Between reps 9 and 12, you
may feel a burning sensation in your triceps, starting with your
elbow and moving up to your shoulder. If you can, continue to
exercise without resting.

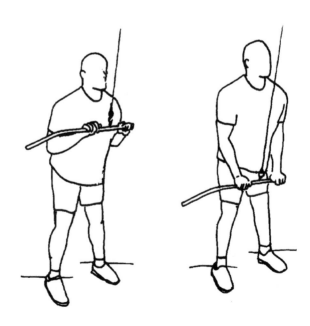

CONCENTRATED BICEPS CURL

What to do:
Sit on a flat bench. Lift the dumbbell with one hand and place the back of the arm (triceps) on the corresponding thigh. To help your balance, place the other hand on the opposite thigh. Slowly raise the weight until your biceps is fully contracted. Then, again slowly, return your arm to the starting position, keeping your elbow slightly bent. Your arm should be in line with your inner thigh and the rest of your body should be as still as possible. If possible, don't rest between reps. Control your movements. Exhale as your raise the weight and inhale as your return to the starting position.

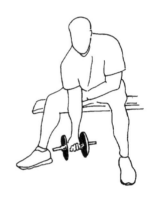

What to expect:
During the first 8 reps be aware of your positioning. Between reps 9 and 12 you may start to feel a burning and a tightening sensation in your biceps.

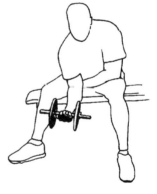

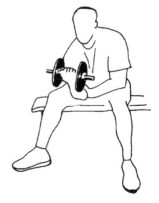

FOREARM BICEPS CURL

What to do:
Sit on flat bench. Lift the dumbbell with both hands and place your arms on the bench with your palms up. Make sure that your wrists are just over the end of the bench. Slowly raise the weight until your forearm is fully contracted. Then, again slowly, return your arm to the starting position while keeping ing your arms on the bench. Your arm should be in line with the bench, as you straddle it, and your body should be as still as possible. Exhale as you raise the weight and inhale as you return to the starting position. Control your movements.

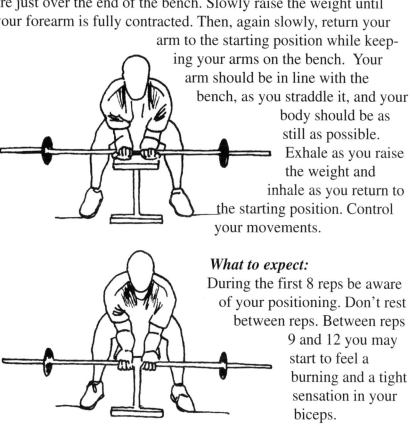

What to expect:
During the first 8 reps be aware of your positioning. Don't rest between reps. Between reps 9 and 12 you may start to feel a burning and a tight sensation in your biceps.

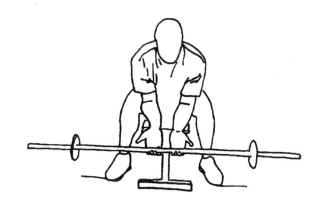

CHAPTER TEN

THE REST OF YOUR LIFE

Anybody can get active. And you have. You are more fit than you were when you started and you know more about yourself. You have reached this point because you were committed to reaching the completion of this book and to feeling better. Now that you've almost reached completion, you may be asking yourself, "What's next? Where do I go from here?" Before we give you specifics about an ongoing program of health, take the time now to look at how your attitude toward exercise may have changed.

Throughout each of the chapters you were asked questions about how you felt before and after your workout. These questions were asked in order for you to become more aware of what factors affected your motivation. Now is the time to go back over your answers and see if you've changed your feeling and thoughts significantly about your workouts. Do you see any changes in your answers?

1. How do you feel before starting your workout?
Count the number of times you answered the following.

_____Motivated   _____ Resigned

_____Discouraged   _____ Anxious

_____Excited   _____ Pressed for time

_____Dreading   _____ Confident

_____Not sure   _____ Ready and willing

_____Clearheaded   _____ Don't want to think about it

How can you change the ones that are consistently negative?

How can you maintain the ones that are consistently positive?

2. How did you feel while you were exercising?
Count the number of times you answered the following.

____ Needed more energy   ____Distracted by negative thoughts

____Could have gone on forever   ____My body really hurt

____Energetic   ____Powerful

____Active   ____Enjoyment

____Fun   ____Invigorated

3. How did you feel after you exercised?
Count the number of times you answered the following.

____ Glad it's over   ____ Dreading the next time

____ Accomplished   ____ Can't wait until next time

____ Successful   ____ I understand its importance

____ Rejuvenated   ____ Wish I'd started this long ago

____ Joyful   ____ I didn't like doing this

Add up your responses in each category. Do you see a pattern of thoughts and feelings? Are you responding more negatively before, during or after your workout? It's for your well-being that you concentrate on why it's important to workout. A good example to keep in mind is:

"A workout is 25% perspiration and 75% determination. Stated another way, it is one part physical exertion and three parts self-discipline. Doing it is easy once you get started. A workout makes you better today than you were yesterday. It strengthens the body, relaxes the mind, and toughens the spirit. When you work out regularly, your problems diminish and your confidence grows.

A workout is a personal triumph over laziness and procrastination. It is the badge of a winner—the mark of an organized goal-oriented person who has taken charge of his or her destiny. A workout is a wise use of time and an investment in excellence. It is a way of preparing for life's challenges and proving to yourself that you have what it takes to do what is necessary.

A workout is a key that helps unlock the door to opportunity and success. Hidden within each of us is an extraordinary force. Physical and mental fitness are the triggers that can release it. A workout is a form of rebirth. When you finish a good workout, you don't simply feel better. You will feel better about yourself."

You also examined the influences in your daily life. These were: expectations, roles, perceptions/attitude, and physical, emotional and social environments. All of these affect your progress toward a healthy lifestyle. As a result of continually writing out your answers to these, you may notice that now they are always in the back of your mind as you go through your day. This is the short term effect of our program. But what about the rest of your life: Indicate which one of the influences have you noticed a pattern of negative or positive behavior while working through *Your Personal Trainer*?

____Expectations   ____Roles

____Physical environment   ____Emotional environment

____Social environment   ____Perceptions

How can you make adjustments in these areas?

Expectations

Roles

Physical environment

Emotional environment

Social environment

Perception/Attitude

You've looked at yourself closely. You know what motivates you and what gets in your way. You know how to set goals and how to strive for them. And most importantly, you've learned to accept yourself.

One of the most important parts of *Your Personal Trainer's* philosophy is that to continue a healthy lifestyle, you must be motivated from within. We didn't offer you the chance to look like someone else, we offer you the chance to be the healthiest you can, and to enjoy your life in the process.

STRUCTURING YOUR EXERCISES FOR LIFE LONG ENJOYMENT

It's important to structure your exercise for long term benefits. To prevent boredom, try these suggestions.

WEEKLY ROUTINES

1. For cardiovascular only, work out every other day for a four-day workout week. Or work out four days in a row, rest on the fifth day, then repeat.

    Workout 1: Cardio only (40 – 60 minute workout)

2. Combine cardiovascular work with muscular strength endurance training workouts. Work out two days, then rest one, work out two more days, then rest two for a four-day workout week. Repeat this pattern. Work out three days, rest one, then repeat this pattern for a six-day workout week.

Workout 2: Cardio (20 – 30 minutes) at the start of each workout

Day 1: Lower body exercises	Day 2: Upper body exercises
Day 3: Rest 24 hours	Day 4: Lower body exercises
Day 5: Upper body exercises	Day 6: Rest
Day 7: Rest	Repeat all days

Choose workouts one and two if:

> ***you need a longer rest time to recuperate***
> ***you haven't exercised in three months or more***
> ***you are just starting for the first time***
> ***you only have an hour a day to devote to exercising***
> ***you want to reduce overeating and stress***

If you can't schedule the same time each day, don't worry. It's more important that you do the work.

Workout 3: Cardio (20-40 minutes) at the start of each workout

Day 1: Legs/abs	Day 2: Back/shoulders/abs
Day 3: Chest/arms/abs	Day 4: Rest 24 hours
Day 5: Legs/abs	Day 6: Back/shoulders/abs
Day 7: Chest/arms/abs	Repeat all days

Although you are resting less with this workout schedule, the benefits of workout three are:

> *you force your body to work at a higher metabolic rate*
> *you reduce fat and increase muscular development*
> *you can change the look of your body faster*

Don't worry if you can't exercise at the same time each day. Varying the times can actually increase the benefits of exercising.

Reflecting on the other benefits of an exercise routine:
> Improved cardiovascular and circulatory systems
> A firmer and more toned body
> Greater mental discipline
> More energy
> An ability to cope with anxiety and tension
> An increased awareness of the close relation between physical and mental functioning
> An enhancement of visualization and concentration skills

Reflecting on the benefits of eating healthfully:
> Optimal food consumption for physical and mental tasks
> Reduction in emotional response eating

Reflecting on the benefits of written exercises:
> Helps you keep an awareness of the influences in daily life
> Helps to think positively
> Helps to achieve goals
> Improves knowledge of positive and negative energy levels
> Gives an overview of what is done each day

We encourage you to take what we have given you and make the necessary changes that fit your future needs. *Your Personal Trainer* is only a foundation on which to build. We hope you will take the information you have received, modify it to suit your needs and develop a long term program for a healthy lifestyle.

FOR LIFE from Your Personal Trainer

AFTERWORD

If you could see me now, you would see a big smile on my face. Why? Because, like myself, you have successfully worked through *Your Personal Trainer*. Just as you have learned, I first had to understand as much as I could about a healthy lifestyle and how I wanted my life to be. I had to look at what motivated me and what my goals were. For me, there was a big difference between knowing what I should want for myself and what I was willing to do. As I was able to define my own needs and desires and what I was willing to act on, I was able to recognize barriers and remove them. This is an approach I've chosen to use for the rest of my life.

I have continued to use this approach to life. I eat healthfully, but don't deprive myself or feel guilty about the foods that are not considered healthy, but taste good to me. Work out, but don't compare my body with an unrealistic look that I know is genetically impossible for me to obtain. I'm working within my body's capacity and have achieved physical balance. I've learned that being able to reflect on how I feel and think on a daily base will also help me achieve mental fitness. Choosing to write to balance negative and positive influences has helped me remove many negative influences that could have caused my life to spin out of balance.

William Kennamore, C.P. T.

In helping write *Your Personal Trainer* I have stressed valuable information that will help you maintain ideal health. Your rewards include feeling physically and emotionally your best, thereby giving yourself the best chance for optimal longevity. For you, just as for the patients in my own practice, I provide this information and guidance to help optimize health and prevent disease. But keep in mind that the medical field is constantly changing. The half life of medical knowledge is considered to be approximately seven years. This means that in seven years half of what we now know to be true will no longer be considered valid.

This fact is exemplified by our change in emphasis toward exercise over the years. When I completed medical school in 1983, physicians recommended primarily aerobic exercise, as strengthening and weight resistance training were felt to add little to one's health. Now through the years we've realized that weight resistance exercises play a critical role in helping maximize the body's metabolic rate, especially for those trying to reduce fat weight. Additionally, stretching exercises keep muscles and joints limber and help prevent injury and arthritis. Both stretching and strengthening should be incorporated along with aerobic exercise to create a balanced program. I'm sure our medical knowledge will evolve further over the coming years. So remember, as part of your healthy lifestyle it's important to keep informed of new and ever changing information.

Jeffrey G. Riopelle, M.D.

ORDERING INFORMATION

YES, I want to increase and maintain my energy and improve my level of fitness! *Your Personal Trainer* available for only $19.95 (price subject to change) each–plus $3.00 shipping and handling.

Please send me: _____ Copies of
Your Personal Trainer @ $19.95 each
_____ CA residents add $1.65 (8.25%) sales tax

Subtotal _____
Postage _____
Grand Total _____

Please allow six to eight weeks for delivery.

NAME _____
ADDRESS_____
CITY _____
STATE _____ZIP_____
PHONE _____

Form of payment:
Check or money order enclosed
(Please make checks payable to: DEMOR)

☐ MASTERCARD   ☐ VISA   ☐ AMEX   ☐ DISCOVER

NAME ON CREDIT CARD _____
ACCOUNT NUMBER _____
EXPIRATION _____
SIGNATURE _____

Mail to: DEMOR, Inc., P. O. Box 393, San Ramon CA 94583

Credit card orders call TOLL FREE:**1-888-2BEFIT6 (223-3486)**